PRAISE FOR *POSITIVELY PRIMAL*

'*Positively Primal* i   estyle. Through
research and discu   ok provides us
with direction on h   res of modern
life. As always, Emr   ...ding, comfort
and support; I know   ...... ume and time again... a well-
balanced and beautifu..., written companion to life.'

Renee McGregor, dietitian and sport nutritionist,
and author of *Training Food*

'I am never happier than when outside, searching for wildlife or
on expeditions. The simplicity to life, the fresh air, the elements
and activity bless us in ways we cannot possibly quantify. I salute
Positively Primal for attempting to bring this ethos to as many people
as possible.'

Steve Backshall, wildlife presenter, naturalist and adventurer

'*Positively Primal* is inspiring and well-researched, showing a depth
of knowledge. Many things in this book are quite remarkable. There
are passages which I plan to share with my clients, a very mature
kind of wisdom on the part of someone who is still young... To read
Emma Woolf's contributions thus is a privilege of its own kind.'

Deanne Jade, psychologist and founder of the
National Centre For Eating Disorders

'This book will inspire you to transform the way you live, and
discover a deeper sense of joy. As the book says, "...do what you can
to change this world for the better and have fun along the way."'

Clea Grady, Veganuary

PRAISE FOR *LETTING GO*

'A practical and heartfelt guide to healing for anyone who has suffered from low self-esteem, a lack of confidence, or disordered eating. Woolf writes with intelligence, wisdom and compassion for a generation of women battling an enduring media onslaught of perfectionism. The fightback continues.'

Rhiannon Lucy Cosslett, *The Vagenda*

'Psychology, philosophy and personal growth marvellously rolled into one, *Letting Go* is a must-read. This book shows us how to develop inner confidence, open new doors, and rediscover joy and meaning in our lives.'

Deanne Jade, psychologist and founder of the
National Centre For Eating Disorders

'*Letting Go* is not about giving up, but about letting freedom in. This brave and personal account shows us that the path to true liberation is through embracing our true selves, however flawed we fear they might be.'

Sally Brampton, author of *Shoot the Damn Dog* and
columnist for *Top Santé* and *Psychologies*

'A timely reminder that though we may take ourselves for granted at times, self-care is a divine responsibility. In Woolf's intimately personal yet relatable voice, *Letting Go* empowers us to accept both the role of wounded and healer.'

Caroline Kent, *Telegraph* journalist

'Gutsy and engaging, *Letting Go* combines research and real-life advice on fulfilling your inner potential and building self-belief... Woolf's latest book is highly recommended.'

Tim Weeks, Olympic trainer

PRAISE FOR *AN APPLE A DAY*

'*An Apple a Day* is the single most important book in my library. I genuinely believe that I am alive because of it. It saved my life.'

Martha Greengrass

'I read *An Apple a Day*, and cried and cried. Reading about the illness in black and white forced me to admit to myself that I did have a problem... Through baring your innermost thoughts and feelings you have given me so much support. Thank you.'

Tessa

'I cannot thank you enough for writing *An Apple a Day*... I could write and write and write forever about all the ways you helped me, but I am going to sit and enjoy the rest of my food now, because of you :)'

Samantha

'Second time reading *An Apple a Day* – honestly the most inspiring thing I've ever read.'

Charlotte (@char_cassels)

'When I read *An Apple a Day*, I finally realised that my struggle was a real one and that I was not alone... Thank you for reminding me that this isn't living. Thank you for reminding me: I want my life back.'

Yasmin

'I first read *An Apple a Day* when I was in my very worst struggle with anorexia, and looking back I can truly say that it was one of the things that saved me. Your words are so real and true... Opening up to the public and media about eating disorders is such an incredibly brave thing to do. I admire you so much. Thank you for everything you do.'

Aine

PRAISE FOR *THE MINISTRY OF THIN*

'Just finished reading *The Ministry of Thin* by @EJWoolf. It strengthened my resolve to be pro-cake, pro-health and pro-happiness. Awesome read.'

@CakeSpy

'It is because of you and your books that you have conveyed to me and thousands of others that I am able to truly believe I am totally, utterly, and undoubtedly worthy of being totally, utterly and beautifully free of my own demons... You have reached out to me without even knowing.'

SV

'I cannot put *The Ministry of Thin* down! It should be on school compulsory reading lists... Inspires a lot of question and debate.'

Emma Louise Vizard (@EmmiLouize)

'Your books *An Apple a Day* and *The Ministry of Thin* have been essential reading in preventing my own relapse while I'm studying at university. Time and again they have stopped me from falling back into that dark, dark place.'

ML

'I loved *The Ministry Of Thin* – I don't believe there's anyone with a better overall grasp of body image issues than Emma Woolf right now.'

Kate Long

'*The Ministry of Thin* is a call to arms – *Fat is a Feminist Issue* for our times.'

Katharine Quarmby, *Newsweek Europe*

POSITIVELY
PRIMAL

POSITIVELY PRIMAL

Summersdale Publishers Ltd
46 West Street
Chichester
West Sussex
PO19 1RP
UK

www.summersdale.com

Printed and bound by CPI Group (UK) Ltd, Croydon, CR0 4YY

ISBN: 978-1-84953-839-8

Substantial discounts on bulk quantities of Summersdale books are available to corporations, professional associations and other organisations. For details contact Nicky Douglas by telephone: +44 (0) 1243 756902, fax: +44 (0) 1243 786300 or email: nicky@summersdale.com.

POSITIVELY
PRIMAL

Finding Health and
Happiness in a Hectic World

EMMA WOOLF

Also by Emma Woolf:

An Apple a Day

The Ministry of Thin

Ways of Escape

Letting Go

Contents

Let us give Nature a chance;
she knows her business better than we do.
Michel de Montaigne

With freedom, books, flowers, and the moon,
who could not be happy?
Oscar Wilde

Introduction

What's It All About?

Modern life can cause us to feel profoundly disconnected from our primal nature. Too often we find ourselves living as we feel we *should*, rather than as we'd like. We eat the food we think we ought to eat, force ourselves through repetitive workouts at the gym, pursue careers which are less than fulfilling and go to work each day with less than a spring in our step. When we turn on the news, we're confronted with terrible events happening around the world: from civil wars and terrorism to famines and natural disasters. Then we look at the damage we're doing to our environment; the relentless airport expansions, road-building and pollution. It's easy to feel powerless and to despair.

Sometimes we even despair about ourselves. We tell ourselves that things would be better if only we were smarter, richer, younger, prettier or thinner. We imagine that other people are happier; we buy and consume more stuff; we look at our bodies in the mirror and dislike what we see. We touch our smartphones more than we touch each other, leaving us lonelier and more disconnected than ever.

What if life could be simpler? What if we could banish fear, obligation and deprivation, and decide to live instead by instinct, joy and kindness? What if we could replace virtual connection with truly meaningful human interaction? What if we could get back in touch with our natural, primal selves and regain that spring in our step?

Do you feel completely in tune with yourself? Can you say that you listen and respond to your body's appetites and desires? Do you trust your physical needs for food and sleep? Do you respond to your instincts for sex and play? Are you comfortable with yourself, at peace in your own skin? Do you feel that your mind and body are in sync?

If you can answer yes to all these questions: congratulations! But many of us cannot. Rates of anxiety, depression, suicide, divorce and loneliness are on the increase, as are eating disorders and obesity. It's not only adults who are affected: an international survey on well-being found that children and adolescents scored among the lowest on levels of self-confidence, body image and happiness. As we enjoy greater wealth, higher living standards, better healthcare and faster technology than at any time in the past, it seems illogical that we should be *less* happy than the generations who went before us.

Positively Primal is a journey of self-discovery, based on ancient philosophy, modern science and common sense, and respect for our individuality, others and the world in which we live. It involves no rules, no restrictive diets, no expensive supplements or equipment – and no deprivation. There are enough rules already in modern life: *Positively Primal* will liberate you from rules. Your primal nature is already within you. You hold the key to becoming happier, calmer and stronger.

There is no doubt that we're yearning for a more natural way of life. From wild swimming to vegetable growing and barefoot running to clean eating, the primal lifestyle is coming into its own. Whether by decluttering or disconnecting, many of us are longing to streamline and simplify. We have reached 'peak stuff', with too many material possessions, and research shows that it's making us ill. Two-thirds of us think we would be better off if we lived more simply and many feel weighed down by their own excess. People who struggle with too much stuff in their homes are more likely to feel stressed, tired and depressed, and have a higher mortality rate. The problem has been dubbed 'stuffocation', and likened to the material equivalent of obesity.

Freed of the junk of our everyday lives, we feel mentally clearer and spiritually lighter. Reducing life to the essentials feels elemental and natural, and it allows us to work out what matters: family, friends, health, the planet; and what doesn't: bank balance, social status, job title, possessions... As well as a resurgence in spirituality and humanism, there is a dawning realisation that, beyond the basics, *more* possessions don't make us *more* satisfied. It's also good for our wallets: buying less reminds us that there is so much more to life than acquiring stuff.

Decluttering our physical surroundings encourages us to live more authentically. Living elementally, in tune with the seasons, makes sense on every level: it's good for our mental and physical health, for our relationships and for the environment. Indeed, our desire to live more minimally is linked to growing environmental awareness about the sheer wastefulness of modern life.

Prehistoric man may seem impossibly remote, but in evolutionary terms, those 20,000 years are a blink of an eye. While few of us would want to go back to living in caves, wearing animal skins and dying in middle age, there is much we can learn from our primal ancestors. They lived in close communion with the Earth, with each other and with their own bodies; they hunted, ate and slept in a more symbiotic cycle with the sun and the seasons.

I'm not the only one to have serious concerns about where our species is heading. For all the amazing benefits of the digital revolution – and there are many – who is really in control these days? The human mind is ingenious and limitless in its capacity for inventiveness, but in the end, humans need more than just faster Wi-Fi, driverless cars and pizzas delivered to our door at the touch of an app. We may live in concrete jungles, but we still need to feel the earth beneath our feet, the rain on our faces and the wind in our hair. We continue to love the wild places and still yearn to get back to nature. Why else would we flock en masse to marvel at the Grand Canyon and to climb mountains so we can wonder at the unspoilt regions of the planet?

More or Less Primal – Your Choice

The beautiful thing about going primal is that it's individual and gradual: the extent to which you make changes is entirely up to you. While I advocate (and personally crave) regular breaks from technology, for example, it's totally your choice to what extent you disconnect, and how often. You could try going offline for a few hours to see how you feel and to begin to experience the benefits; a few hours could then become a day or even a whole weekend. The same goes for primal eating: you could have meat-free days, or experiment with vegetarian recipes, but it doesn't need to happen all at once.

Being positively primal isn't all or nothing. Chances are, the more opportunities you find to reconnect with yourself, with real food and the world around you, the more you'll enjoy it. But it's a process which can happily co-exist with modern life: take it slow and enjoy the journey, rather than launching yourself into a punitive regime.

Going primal is also a virtuous circle. It's about developing a more intuitive relationship with the world around us, as well as with ourselves. Concern for our fragile planet is increasing, with millions of us facing up to the fact that oil, coal and gas are finite resources, and we need to find another way. What is infinite, of course, are those natural, renewable sources of energy: wind, sea and solar.

To these sources of renewable energy, I would add human ingenuity, positivity and kindness. Living more primally means thinking seriously about how we consume, and how we can reuse more and waste less.

Going primal is also economical: it involves no expensive equipment, ingredients or gym memberships. And that's precisely the point. The more you're using your body and your natural surroundings – to work out, to travel, to feed yourself – the more primal you become. Consuming less meat, turning down your heating, walking and cycling more? Of course you're going to look and feel a million times better! It's a win-win situation – and, I promise you, it's pain-free.

Ditch the Rules

As anyone who has ever tried a strict diet knows, rules are for fools. How many of us start the new year with a list of resolutions, a pristine pair of trainers or a cupboard full of superfood powders and potions? Mostly, this induces a feeling of obligation and deprivation: I *must* go running five mornings a week, I *must* drink three green juices a day and I *must not* eat chocolate or cake.

On your primal journey, there are no rules: you can be a meat-eater or a vegetarian, a wine-lover or teetotal, super-sporty or not-so-active, a leftie environmentalist or a free-market capitalist – or anything in between. The journey is about rediscovering your creative side, finding solutions to personal challenges, and exploring your own curiosity and strength. It's not about following rules.

While eating fresh produce and getting active will lead to a healthier – and probably fitter – you, *Positively Primal* is emphatically not about weight loss. We won't be focusing on shedding pounds, and the phrase 'drop a dress size' will not pass my lips. If you want to feel happier and stronger, this is the book for you; if you just want to get thin, not so much.

When you're at peace in your own skin, with fulfilling work and good relationships, everything else falls into place. That could well include self-esteem, body issues and disordered eating, but this book is not about how you look or what you weigh. It focuses on how you feel and who you are; it's about valuing your body, rather than comparing it to others or measuring how it falls short.

Back to the Future

On your journey towards – or back to – a more primal existence, we'll explore every aspect of physical and mental well-being. We'll look at eating, exercising, working and playing in a more primal way. And we'll look at thoughts and emotions, our relationships with others, and how to feel more in tune with the seasons and the world around us. We'll look at Ayurveda, the ancient Indian science of well-being, and how to work out your individual 'dosha' type. Along the way we'll explore the evidence for the benefits of going primal, by way of research and real-life stories, tips and advice from a range of nutritional, fitness, scientific and spiritual experts and professionals.

I recently went to see the Indian mystic Sadhguru speak in London. At the end of his talk he asked this simple question:

'Did the sun rise and did you wake up this morning?'

Like the rest of the audience, I thought: *of course the sun rose. Of course I woke up… So what?*

Yes, *so what?* Of course you woke up today, since you're reading this book. But stop to consider for a moment: approximately one million people around the world die each day. That's a million people who did not wake up this morning, who will never see another sunrise

– to say nothing of the millions of bereaved families and friends they leave behind. Today dawned, just as it should, maybe without you even noticing. The sun did not collide with another planet or explode in a ball of flames. You did not die, and neither (I hope) did anyone you love.

Reflecting on this miracle made me feel ashamed of my occasional grumpiness on waking. Really, no day should be a 'bad day' – remember, whatever else happens, you're alive. This is what the primal approach is all about: finding simple pleasure in the everyday.

Whether you already live a perfectly primal lifestyle, or these are your first steps, I hope you'll find it fulfilling. With the pace and impersonality of modern existence, it can be easy to feel anxious, disconnected or simply burnt out. On this primal journey, you'll rediscover your natural *joie de vivre*, the capacity for human joy that lies within every one of us. Taking a primal path allows you to enjoy your health through activity and adventure, to tune into your instincts and appetites, and to live in harmony with the natural world. I can't promise you a new body in seven days but I can help you discover a new mindset which will last a lifetime. Remember: the main things are to embrace the primal journey, to do what you can to change this world for the better, and to have fun along the way.

Chapter 1
Primal Mindset

> ❝ *Piglet noticed that even though he had a Very Small Heart, it could hold a rather large amount of Gratitude.* ❞
> **A. A. Milne, *Winnie-the-Pooh***

There are times in everyone's life when things get tough or go off-course, from relationships to work or health. Maybe you feel lost or lonely, demoralised or directionless. Perhaps you think everyone else is happier and more successful than you are. When these times come, as they will for us all, remember that you are not as powerless as you feel. Even when you cannot change the situation, you can modify the way you think about it and react to it. It really is remarkable what a difference our minds can make.

One of the first and most powerful decisions you can make is not to be a victim of circumstance. Negative human habits aren't easy to change – we've all been guilty of complaining and comparing, holding grudges or feeling hard done by – but persistence and determination will get you a long way. Whatever happens, you can choose simply to remain positive, find a bright side and count your blessings, no matter how great the challenges. Gratitude and positivity are at the very heart of the primal mindset.

Less Attitude, More Gratitude

Gratitude is on the up and up. Hot on the heels of the mindfulness trend, gratitude is all over social media, with the obligatory hashtags: #blessed, #humbled, #grateful. We may sneer at the faux-humility and the humblebrags, but we shouldn't dismiss the power of gratitude. It is, quite simply, one of the most valuable habits you can take up.

Gratitude transforms uncertainty into clarity, bitterness into happiness and regret into joy. It's also good for our mental and physical health. A study reported by the American Psychological Association found that more gratitude was associated with 'better mood, better sleep, less fatigue and lower levels of inflammatory biomarkers related to cardiac health'. Psychologists also believe it may help in the prevention and treatment of clinical depression.

We're often told that learning to live in the present moment, and practising mindfulness, increases our potential for happiness. In a similar way, being grateful adds to the joy we feel. And while mindfulness isn't an easy skill to master, gratitude couldn't be simpler. It requires nothing but an open heart and open eyes, because the good is already there, all around us in our lives. It involves no complicated system of skills or beliefs: it's simply saying thank you for what you already have. No matter how hard things get, keep returning to that simple fact: this is a life of abundance and good fortune. Counting your blessings strengthens the gratitude muscle and enriches daily life.

Remember: it's not happiness that makes us grateful, but gratefulness that makes us happy.

Lucky You

When I say that this is a life of 'abundance', I really mean it. Right now, more than 1.3 billion people worldwide live in extreme poverty, surviving on less than $1.25 a day. Also, 805 million people do not have enough food to eat, more than 750 million people lack access to clean drinking water and approximately 1.6 billion people live without electricity.

Pause for a moment, and look at what you're doing: reading this book, perhaps using the Internet, sipping a coffee, warm and fed, with clothes on your back and a roof over your head. There are electric lights around you, and hot and cold running water in the taps. No matter what your individual circumstances, yours is a life of tremendous good luck and abundance, even riches.

Reasons to Be Grateful

Gratitude has been proven to beget more gratitude: if you spend a few moments tuning in to the great things in your life, you tend to notice them more throughout the rest of your day.

Gratitude is liberating. Being thankful is stronger than anger, regret or negativity. When you can say 'thank you for the experience', you're able to forgive and move on.

Gratitude makes you see that what you have right now is enough. You never really need more than what you have in the present moment. Inhabit this moment, and savour it.

If you're in a dark place, remember that nothing stays the same forever. Life will inevitably surprise you again in some unimaginable way. Don't assume that you're stuck with the way things are right now. You aren't: life can, and will, change in an instant.

How to Get Started

Make your gratitude all-inclusive. Appreciate everything and everyone in your life. Give thanks for the lessons you've learned, the people you've met and the love you've felt.

Give back. When a person or organisation has helped you in some way, try to return the favour, or at least acknowledge their impact on your life. Writing thank-you cards may be old-fashioned, but so what? A box of chocolates, a bunch of flowers, a hug or a kind word never disappoints!

Don't look back in anger. Ban *what-ifs* and *if-onlys* from your vocabulary. Just because something doesn't last forever, that doesn't mean it wasn't good while it lasted. Replace regret with a sense of wonder.

Let go of control: you cannot control what happens; you can only live for each moment. When you appreciate the present, you'll find yourself worrying less about the past and the future.

Keep it simple, keep it primal. If you're struggling to feel positive (and we all do sometimes), start with the simplest things: the grass between your toes, the sun on your face, the wind in your hair and the rain on your skin. We live in an amazing world; there is always something to be grateful for.

Tracking Your Gratitude

Most positive-thinking experts recommend keeping a daily journal in which to record special moments or reasons to be happy and grateful. While I agree with the power of thinking thankfully, I don't believe you have to write it in a journal. Keeping a permanent list makes me feel as though I should be coming up with profound events or emotions to be recorded for all time, different every day. In fact, gratitude can and should be just the opposite: simple moments of pleasure in the everyday.

A disposable list, such as a Post-it note or the back of a receipt which you can chuck away, can feel more liberating. I often scribble my gratitude moments on the back of my hand, where I'll see it for a few hours before it gets washed off. See what works for you: transient jottings of those daily smiles can be just as powerful as a formal journal.

For example, today my three 'gratitude moments' were: sipping freshly brewed coffee, having a lane to myself during my morning swim, and the rain stopping and the sun finally coming out: nothing profound! They may well be similar most days, if nothing more spectacular happens in my life... And that's fine too.

From Anger to Thankfulness

Modern life is filled with stressors: slow broadband, delayed trains, office politics... It can be easy to find yourself clenched with rage when the day has barely begun. Our default responses range from irritation to indignation, and sometimes even public outbursts. The gratitude mindset works along similar principles to mindfulness: you observe and absorb events around you, rather than rushing straight to those immediate angry reactions.

Negative, cynical, dissatisfied, critical: recognise any of these attitudes in yourself? I do, perhaps on a daily basis! I can become impatient too quickly and criticise others too easily. This doesn't make me a bad person, but it's not a relaxing way to live. We're all prone to these cycles of negativity so try to catch yourself whenever yours start.

The primal gratitude mindset is a powerful way of pausing the habitual cycle of negative thinking. Here are a few simple mind-changers.

Rather than tweeting about the transport chaos or gridlocked traffic, why not stare out of the window at the landscape? It could be suburban back gardens, a vibrant cityscape or rolling green fields. Absorb yourself in that view.

When a partner, friend or family member irritates you, take a deep breath and think about how lucky you are to have met them. Imagine your life without them in it. Put minor niggles out of your mind and focus instead on the things that you both enjoy. Making them smile will cheer you both up.

If the queues in the sandwich shop are long, use the free time for some deep breathing. You could gaze at the different colours, textures and tastes of the food on offer. Invent new sandwich combinations in your mind. You could even strike up a conversation with the person next to you.

If things are difficult at the office, try to see the broader picture. We don't get to choose our colleagues – and workplaces can be claustrophobic – but learning to deal with others is a valuable life skill. Stay calm and stay courteous. If you feel yourself getting irritated, go for a walk at lunchtime or remove yourself from the situation. If all else fails, offer to make tea for everyone or bring in a cake – sweet things will soften even the hardest of hearts, and a kind offer can diffuse workplace tension.

Various apps can send gratitude reminders directly to your phone. They prompt you to think of a few things that you're grateful for every day, for example, and even to take pictures of them to deepen your appreciation of the moment. If you find yourself getting swept up in the rush and routine of everyday life, these can be a useful reminder to slow down and count your blessings.

Positive and Primal

Practising positivity is an essential aspect of maintaining a happy, primal mindset. Thinking and behaving positively creates a virtuous cycle which strengthens your resilience through the tough times, helps you to support others, and boosts your own well-being and success. Put simply, it's deciding to look on the bright side.

Is it really a decision? I believe it is. Optimism (or pessimism) is a choice which is entirely within your grasp. While we cannot always control what events life throws at us, we can decide how we react to them. We all know people who have suffered undeserved life traumas, illness or bereavements, and still remain sunny. Think of the stories of Holocaust survivors, or veterans of the First and Second World Wars, helping others in the same desperate situation, sharing their meagre rations, putting others first. Some of the most compassionate, altruistic people I know have endured tragedy in their lives – and their kindness has helped them and those around them to survive.

Most of us, fortunately, will never experience such horrors, but we all go through ups and downs. And when we're down, it's really worth focusing on the light at the end of the tunnel: research has shown that optimists live longer, healthier and happier lives. Some of us are naturally more upbeat, while others are more pessimistic (I can be rather Eeyorish myself) but we mustn't allow random everyday events to plunge us into melancholy. There *are* silver linings in every black cloud.

Accentuate the Positive

Whether it's taking a few moments for gratitude every night or telling the people close to you how much you value them, there are easy ways to boost your positivity. Like any muscle, the more you think positive, the stronger this habit becomes.

Like attracts like: adopting a positive, welcoming attitude to what you have will attract more positivity into your life.

Positivity doesn't have to be saccharine or fake; it simply means appreciating good friends, good food and good times.

Make a conscious decision to cherish the good bits (and endure the bad bits) in your life. Practise grace under pressure, whatever comes your way, and graciousness with others, whatever they do or say.

Forgiveness

As well as practising positivity, we also need to learn to forgive. No matter how positively we think and behave, no matter how carefully we plan for the future, sometimes things just go wrong.

We live in an uncertain world, at a time of global pandemics, terrorism and natural disasters. On a personal level too, life can be uncontrollable. It could be a small blip, such as a row with your boss or a minor car scrape, or it could be serious and life-changing such as divorce, bereavement or a terrible accident. There is no way to avoid the unexpected in life – but there is one skill you can master: the human, primal, simple act of forgiveness.

1. The past is the past. Whatever has happened has happened. You can't change that; you can only control how you act in the present, and how you plan for the future. Forgiveness is about cleansing the slate and moving forward. It's incredibly hard – but crucial.

2. Just do it. Sometimes you need to forgive yourself, sometimes you need to forgive others and sometimes, say in the event of a natural disaster, you don't even know who to forgive. There is

still great power in the act of forgiveness, because it means letting go of fault, blame and regret.

3. Be aware of your thoughts and feelings: mindfulness is very helpful in the process of forgiveness. You won't always have control over your thoughts, but be aware of them, watch them come and go. When they're negative and painful, acknowledge this to yourself. When your feelings start to change, maybe even improve, acknowledge this too. Separate yourself from the maelstrom of emotions.

4. Success is the best revenge. If someone has hurt or mistreated you, leave it behind. Don't waste time hating them or trying to get your own back. Choose to be positive rather than negative in the face of adversity. You're not to blame for their bad behaviour, so don't dwell on it. Forget them, move on and find kinder, better people to spend your life with.

5. Accept that everyone screws up. Yes, everyone! Learning to forgive yourself and others means learning not to sweat the small stuff. Your past, my past, all our pasts are littered with mistakes – things we shouldn't have said and done and thought and bought... The only reason for dwelling on those mistakes is to learn from them. Build on your past, using those errors as stepping stones for future growth. Learning to forget can be as important as leaning to forgive.

Compare and Despair

Forgiving *more* is part of the primal journey – and so is comparing *less*. In our fast-paced, highly visual and fiercely competitive culture, we're all prone to the 'compare and despair' syndrome. We fail to appreciate our own achievements, even if we've worked damn hard for them, because there's always the next big thing: you finally get the promotion you've been working for, or the flat or car you've been saving for, but you barely appreciate it, because you're aware of still being several steps behind other people. Don't forget to stop and savour the experience: there is absolutely nothing wrong with rejoicing in your own success.

Appreciating yourself is as important as appreciating others. You can just decide, right now, to value who and what you are. Choose to challenge that hyper-critical inner voice whenever it pipes up, and to turn insecurity and envy into pride and thankfulness.

There are so many opportunities to feel grateful and proud of yourself: in the career or life goals you've achieved, the personal challenges you've overcome, or in the relationships you've created. Do you think that our primal ancestors spent their lives wracked with self-doubt? Take a robust attitude to your own strengths and weaknesses: we all have talents and we all have shortcomings – so what?

In order to value yourself – and participate more fully in your own life – you need to give up a few bad habits:

- constant comparison with others
- feeling hard done by or inadequate
- labelling yourself as a victim
- feeling inferior or unworthy
- bitching about others
- criticising or blaming yourself.

Many of these habits are so deeply ingrained we don't even notice them. Researchers have found, for example, that women have an average of 30 negative body thoughts in a single day. Comparing ourselves to others, trying to 'keep up with the Joneses' is an unfortunate aspect of modern life, as is bitching about others. In reality, you don't need to attack others in order to feel better about yourself. So stop undermining other people, and stop criticising yourself.

Once again, like attracts like. When you're able to appreciate your own qualities, you'll become more able to appreciate others. Just as the gratitude mindset reminds you to count your blessings and appreciate the good in your life, it will also allow you to appreciate your own achievements and value yourself.

Gaining this inner confidence makes you more generous and tolerant towards others. Life isn't a zero-sum game: we can all have strengths and talents, and they don't need to cancel each other out. Unlike a competition or a race, there isn't just one winner.

Of course, gratitude isn't a cure-all: not everything is within your control. Sometimes you want to change a situation but you can't, and that's life. In fact, a lot of what happens will be out of your control: random events, accidents, illness, those intangibles, such as good luck and bad luck, the feelings and reactions of others... The list goes on. As Viktor Frankl, author of *Man's Search for Meaning*, and a Holocaust survivor, writes: 'The last of one's freedoms is to choose one's attitude in any given circumstance.'

Frankl faced unimaginable horrors, far worse than anything most of us will ever encounter. His words are a reminder that, although you cannot control the situation, you can choose how you respond. Learning to adapt your attitude is essential to dealing with whatever life throws at you, and a core aspect of the primal mindset. It means finding an upside in any bad situation – and there *is* always an upside, no matter how desperate it feels.

Learn from Survivors

Hopefully, you're going to live a long life, full of interesting and unexpected events. In the decades ahead, it's inevitable that you'll meet a lot of different people, experience many adventures, learn many lessons... and face some adversities. The anticipation of tough times can be even more frightening than the reality: *how would I cope if someone in my family died?* we think, or *what if I lost my job or my home?*

The fact is, you will cope – we all cope. And this is where you can learn from others. Finding role models when you don't feel strong enough is essential. So many others have faced illness, heartbreak, personal calamity, life-changing accidents, and so on, and survived.

Watch the movie *Touching the Void*, or read Katie Piper's memoir *Beautiful* or *A Grief Observed* by C. S. Lewis. Talk to older friends or your grandparents. When you reflect on how others have faced loss and dragged themselves up from rock bottom, it reminds you that you're not alone.

The Buddhist monk and mindfulness guru Andy Puddicombe has some great ideas on how to counter negative thoughts when they arise. He asks us to tune into our daily 'mind chatter' and check whether it is healthy or unkind: 'If you said the same thing to a close friend, how would you expect them to react? Likewise, if they said the same thing, or spoke in that tone of voice, to you, how would it make you feel?' (www.headspace.com)

If this daily 'mind chatter' is routinely negative, Puddicombe asks you to soften up. After all, if you wouldn't snap at a friend like that, constantly criticise or point out faults, why do it to yourself? Being able to take an outside perspective on your inner self-talk is an essential part of building a positive, constructive relationship with yourself.

Growing, Not Fixed

Whatever situation you're in right now, whoever you are and however you feel, things can change. You are growing, not fixed.

The US social psychologist Carol Dweck has formulated a theory of intelligence that she calls the 'growth mindset'. Based on her years of research into motivation, learning and personality development, she argues that individuals with a 'fixed mindset' tend to fear failure and avoid risk, whereas individuals with a 'growth mindset' are open to learning and improving. She explains:

66 *In a fixed mindset students believe their basic abilities,*
their intelligence, their talents, are just fixed traits.
They have a certain amount and that's that, and then their
goal becomes to look smart all the time and never look dumb.
In a growth mindset students understand that their talents
and abilities can be developed through effort, good teaching
and persistence. They don't necessarily think everyone's the
same or anyone can be Einstein, but they believe everyone
can get smarter if they work at it. 99

Dweck's theory has been a powerful educational tool, encouraging children to keep learning and pushing the boundaries, and guiding teachers on how to praise and develop pupils as they grow. Originally designed with students in mind, the growth mindset is applicable to us all. From a young age, and increasingly as we specialise through school and university subject choices, we tend to narrow down our options. Parents refer to us as the 'clever one' or the 'sporty one' and these early labels tend to stick with us.

Do you recognise any of the following statements?

“ I can't draw to save my life. ”

“ My brother is the brainy one in our family. ”

“ I'm fine with people one-on-one, but terrible with large groups. ”

“ I never did get the hang of maths. ”

“ I'm really unsporty, but that's OK – you can't be good at everything. ”

“ I'm just not a languages person. ”

Here's a revolutionary thought: what if you've changed since you were bottom of your maths class? Could your running have improved since the day you came last in the egg and spoon race in junior school? What if you're now quite good at languages, but you just haven't tried? I'm quite different to how I was at seven years old, and I bet you are too.

It's also important to separate events or 'skills' from who you are as an individual. Too often we confuse what we do with who we are; we measure our self-worth by what we achieve in the outside world. In reality, exams or promotions are only external events. Rejoice in your success, by all means, but keep it in perspective. Losing a race or failing an exam doesn't make you a failure; being good or bad at maths or languages doesn't define you as a person.

The growth mindset is deeply primal, because it's a reminder that every one of us is adaptable, resilient and full of potential. Perhaps you never got the hang of the high jump, algebraic equations or oil painting, but your daily life is full of physical agility, mathematical calculations and moments of creativity! Remember that the best predictor of success isn't past failure but determination, resilience and hard work. The growth mindset reminds you that your abilities and strengths are growing, not fixed; it gives you the confidence to try.

Stay Playful

The one thing that hasn't changed since you were a child is that you still need to play.

'The opposite of play isn't work; it's depression,' says Dr Stuart Brown, founder of the National Institute for Play. As children, play teaches us about positive and negative emotions; we learn about risk-taking, trust, ambiguity, rejection, teamwork and joy. It expands our brains, it's the foundation of relationships, it increases resilience and it develops co-operation. Play can break down prejudice, hatred and intolerance. It helps us to discover more about ourselves: our creative potential, our imagination, our fear and courage.

And it's not just for the young: humans (and primates) go on playing throughout life. Play is necessary for the healthy adult functioning of both body and soul. The benefits of physical exercise are well documented, so playing active games will also bring you the same benefits: it strengthens the heart, stimulates endorphins, improves sleep, and burns off the hormones, sugars and fats released in the bloodstream as a result of stress.

Play also strengthens our cognitive and psychological well-being. There is increasing evidence that intellectually stimulating activities, such as crosswords and Sudoku, can lower the risk of developing dementia and Alzheimer's disease. Intellectual games exercise the mind, just as physical games exercise the body. The researcher Cale Magnuson of the University of Illinois explains: 'To not play puts an individual at risk for many detrimental aging processes.' A lack of physical and mental activity increases the likelihood of developing chronic conditions including diabetes, cancers, obesity and stroke. Play is also beneficial for relationships: having fun together keeps couples emotionally and physically close. Just as with children, recreation, team sports and organised events among adults help to forge community cohesion and build strong social networks.

Without the playful impulse we would have no games, no films, no fashion, no flirtation, no music festivals, no fiction, no sport and no fantasy. Brown calls play 'one of the most advanced methods nature has invented to allow a complex brain to create itself'. If we don't play, we miss out on a positive outlet for negative emotions and daily frustrations. Whether it's meeting a friend for a game of squash, challenging yourself to try a dance class, experimenting with watercolours or writing a short story, give yourself the opportunity to be playful. Be creative, be adventurous and have fun: a life without play isn't worth living.

The Importance of Doing Nothing

As we've seen, play is essential on many levels: physical, psychological and social. Developmental psychologists emphasise the importance of free, unstructured playtime for children in encouraging them to use their imaginations and build creativity. Similarly, adults benefit from unstructured time when we're not doing anything in particular. This kind of aimless downtime allows your mind to wander and your brain to recharge. Indeed, boredom can be a positive experience, motivating us to change the status quo by throwing in a tedious job or relationship, selling up to go travelling or making a fresh start. Without that sense of ennui, we might never realise that life could be different.

Don't over-schedule your life: remember that those resting periods are often the ones when you come up with great ideas or solutions to niggling problems. Think of Archimedes in his bath or Newton under the apple tree and reclaim your right to be idle. Pondering, wandering and daydreaming are positive and primal.

Bend, Don't Break

Just as you keep your body agile and your mind active, you need to keep your attitude flexible. It's unsettling to acknowledge this but nothing in life is guaranteed: not your job, your relationship or your health. Imagine you're made redundant, your partner walks out and you get diagnosed with an incurable disease: what are you going to do? A weak person might simply lie down and give up.

Well, not really. None of us do that – because we're stronger, in the end, than we give ourselves credit for. Human beings, even the least likely among us, have an amazing capacity to just keep going. I remember my grandmother, who used to moan and grumble at the slightest daily inconvenience, being transformed during the final months of her life. She battled cancer with courage and grace: through the worst pain, I never once heard her complain. In the most extreme circumstances, even when dying, humans find this inner fortitude to draw upon. Our positive, primal strength cannot keep us alive forever, but it gives us the bravery to face whatever happens.

With flexibility comes resilience. When life doesn't go the way you plan, not only do you need to adjust your mindset, but you also need to be strong. This is otherwise known as 'bloody-mindedness' – the all-important decision that, whatever happens, you are not going to let this destroy you.

Sometimes, as in Jessica's case, we don't even realise how resilient we are.

> **Jessica, 45:** Three years ago my husband told me he was gay and left me for another man. My entire world collapsed – honestly, I was living in some kind of nightmare. Because of having two young children, though, I *didn't* collapse – I suppose I couldn't. The first 12 months were a blur; I was just looking after the children, feeding them and getting them to school and going to work, doing the shopping, in this fog of pain. I was just putting one foot in front of the other – and in the end, that got me through.

During a crisis, focus on the essentials, and don't worry if standards slip. So you've fed the kids pasta for three nights in a row, the house is a mess, you haven't ironed your shirt for work and your roots need doing... So what? Keeping it primal is about working out what really matters: in Jessica's case, her marriage was imploding but the children were safe and fed. In tough times, adopting this primal mindset is incredibly helpful: ask yourself, what really matters right now? Work out what this is – your health, paying the rent, staying sane – and leave the rest to take care of itself.

Bravery

Jessica didn't have a choice in the collapse of her marriage, but she had a choice in her response. Although it probably didn't feel like it at the time, her decision to carry on shopping, working, mothering and breathing was brave.

Bravery was a pre-requisite of primal survival: for cavemen and women it was a matter of life and death. The risks you face are different to those Palaeolithic perils – more social and reputational risks, less physical danger – but bravery is still bravery, whether it takes the form of confronting a herd of wildebeest or standing up in front of a roomful of colleagues. You are courageous every time you do something which scares you, challenges you or makes you doubt your own ability to cope.

Primal man did not have a choice about risking life and limb to survive. It's worth reminding yourself that in most situations you do have a choice. However, if you consistently choose not to risk anything, life will be pretty boring. You can risk your pride and your reputation – or you can just stay home in your onesie and never do anything brave. It's up to you.

How to Strengthen Your Primal Backbone

- Accept that fear is part of life (everyone feels it).

- Reframe threats as challenges, opportunities to grow. You're not scared; you're excited.

- The perfectionist mindset is exceedingly self-limiting. If you never make mistakes, you will never learn. Embrace failure as an opportunity to improve.

Count down. When I get super-nervous about a forthcoming event, I tell myself: 'In 24 hours this will be over.'

Keep things in perspective: it's easy to let minor fears (e.g. public speaking) rage out of control. It's nerve-wracking, but it's not life-and-death.

Stay primal: what *really* matters? Health and home, family and friends, food and water. If you have all those things, you're doing fine.

Be bullish and brave – ask yourself: what's the absolute worst thing that could happen? But don't catastrophize. The likelihood is that everything won't go wrong.

Try this mantra: 'Everything will be okay in the end. If it's not okay, it's not the end.' (John Lennon)

Breathe: deep breathing slows your heart rate, supplies oxygen to your anxious brain, calms you down and clears your mind.

And remember: whatever happens, you'll be OK.

Stress Less

In modern life, stress is worn as a badge of honour. Like being too busy to sleep or eat, being highly stressed is equated with being powerful and important. Resting is a sign of weakness, and asking for time off is out of the question. We keep going until things get better, or worse, or until we collapse.

However, the more we understand about stress on a physiological level, the more it becomes obvious that this is wrong. Insufficient sleep, excessive caffeine intake, irregular eating and, above all, prolonged stress, are known to be highly damaging to the human organism. Our bodies can cope with short bursts of stress, danger or risk, but we're not designed to handle it in the long term. Being wired all the time takes its toll.

Here's how the body responds to stress.

↓ The adrenal glands, just above the kidneys, begin to produce hormones.

↓ Initially, they pump out adrenalin and noradrenaline to keep the body alert and focused.

↓ Then they pump out cortisol, which converts protein to energy and releases stored sugar, *glycogen*, so we have the fuel needed to respond quickly.

↓ This adrenal response triggers the so-called 'fight or flight' response. Heart and respiratory rates, blood pressure and energy increase, muscles tense, our senses become heightened, and we get ready to escape or to fight back.

↓ The adrenal glands become over-burdened when chronic stress repeatedly forces them to sustain high levels of cortisol. They struggle to regulate hormones, and excess levels of cortisol may damage healthy tissue. Also, high levels of circulating cortisol encourage the body to store excess fat in the abdominal area, rather than on the hips, which is particularly unhealthy for women. The resulting belly fat is a sort of a protective cushion around the middle which, unlike the fat around hips and thighs, is visceral, wrapped around the organs deep inside the body, and it's dangerous. It has been linked to type 2 diabetes, cancer – particularly breast cancer – and even Alzheimer's disease. Excessive cortisol also plays havoc with your appetite, which again leads to weight gain around the middle. In men it can also lead to lower testosterone.

↓ On a day-to-day basis, you may feel constantly exhausted and reliant on stimulants such as caffeine, sugar or alcohol to get you through. Adrenal fatigue may set in, causing weight gain, insomnia, confusion, depression, cravings and mood swings. Extreme stress can cause stroke, heart disease and even death.

Learn to Say No

On top of the regular external sources of stress – traffic, work, bills – there are many stressors that we bring upon ourselves. They often stem from that 'superwoman' (and it *is* usually women) foible of trying to please everyone. You know what happens next: your diary is full of things you don't want to do and you end up stressed out, exhausted or ill.

Many invitations or requests could be politely declined – and think of what you could do with all that free time. Aim for at least three evenings a week when you're not obliged to do anything or be anywhere: no meetings at your child's school, no drinks after work, and so on. Use the time for you, whether that's for some gentle yoga, reading or cooking. Better yet, give yourself an entire weekend off to simply relax and potter.

In order to say 'no' assertively, keep it simple: don't over-apologise, try to be constructive. For example, if a friend wants to talk when you're facing a looming deadline, suggest a time later that evening when you could ring her back. Or if you're asked to help out with a project, suggest other people who might have more time and would welcome the experience. Above all, don't feel guilty: remind yourself that there will always be others who can take on the work.

Learning to say no (politely) is transformative. Not only will it make you calmer and happier, but you'll also be more enthusiastic and efficient when you do get involved. Making time in your life to unwind, de-stress and relax should be a priority, not a luxury or a source of guilt. Stress shouldn't be perceived as a badge of honour but as a serious risk to your health. Remember the primal mindset and slow down. Focus on what's really important, such as the people who matter, and your own health. Taking stress seriously means giving your body the care it needs.

Trust Your Gut

There's a reason why the gut is known as the second brain. Thousands of years before self-help books were invented, and long before psychotherapy, relationship counsellors, life coaches and careers advisors were around, primal humans relied on their bodies to work out what to do. That thing we casually refer to as 'gut instinct' is one of the most important tools we have. This is because our intestines and our emotions are intimately linked. There are a huge amount of nerve connections in the gut. The microbes in the gut pick up chemicals to give the brain signals, so the gut makes neurochemicals, which then create and affect emotions. Instead of weighing up the options or seeking expert advice, sometimes our bodies can be our best guide: just tune in to that 'gut feeling'. From danger radar to stress detector, the humble gut can be a powerful, sometimes life-saving, messenger.

In this Internet age, we're often surrounded by too much information and too many competing opinions. Malcom Gladwell, author of *Blink*, calls this 'analysis paralysis'. He advocates simplifying the decision-making process: 'If the big picture is clear enough, then decide from the big picture without using a magnifying glass.' Learning to listen to – and trust – our gut takes practice, but over time it can become a valuable and reliable guide. We can develop our gut instinct in a couple of simple ways.

Primal decision-making

We assume we should make decisions with our brains, but our bodies are powerful decision-makers too. Choose a situation in which you're wavering between two options.

⚫ First of all, think about one side, for example: 'I want to go back to university and retrain for a completely new career.' While you're pondering this, notice the sensation in your gut. Do you feel a tightening, a gripping feeling? Or softening, spaciousness and warmth? Do you feel comfortable or uneasy?

⚫ Now shift to the other side of the issue: 'I am happy to stick with my current career for the rest of my working life.' Again, tune in to how your gut feels and what kind of thoughts arise. You may not get a definite answer at first, but the more you listen to your body, the more you'll develop a clear gut sense. It's not about right and wrong; it's about which decision *feels* right.

Danger radar

The danger radar was essential to our primal ancestors. Gut feelings also help you to work out whether a person or situation is good or bad for you.

Think back to a time when someone or something made you feel upset or unsettled (even if you're not sure why). Recall that difficult experience and notice what happens in your body. Do you feel tense or relaxed, comfortable or uncomfortable? Is there a knot in your stomach, a lump in your throat? Practise being aware of how your body reacts physically to thoughts and situations. Although you don't always have to act on them, these are important signals.

The gut is also an excellent barometer of stress. Next time you feel anxious or uneasy, try a simple visualisation exercise. Find a memory or place that is special to you, such as walking beside the sea or playing your favourite song. Whatever comes to mind, focus on the details that make this meaningful: the sounds, colours, textures or smells. As you visualise this 'happy' time or place, you'll feel your gut becoming softer and your body more relaxed.

Keeping That Healthy Mindset

'Mens sana in corpore sano' is a Latin saying, meaning a sound mind in a sound body. In order to have a healthy mind, you need a healthy body: they're inextricably linked. How you consciously act affects how you unconsciously think and feel. Every one of your regular activities, from eating to working to exercising to sleeping, has an impact on how you feel and function. Good habits are the building blocks for a good life.

Many of us spend a lot of time looking for the ultimate secret of health and happiness, often wondering what other people know that we don't. In truth, although there is no single, magic secret, we can all boost our well-being in simple ways.

Here are a few 'mind and body' actions that healthy people do on a regular basis. They are practical, proactive and positive.

Cycle anywhere. Get an old bike and cycle to work, to the shops, around the park. Cycling is clean, green and cheap, and it helps to maintain a healthy weight. After smoking, obesity is the most avoidable cause of cancer (Cancer Research study, 2015) so it makes sense to build everyday activity into your life.

Stand up for your health. Research shows that standing instead of sitting has measurable benefits. Standing up for meetings, walking in your lunch break, mowing the lawn, getting off the bus a few stops early... There are endless ways to stay on your toes.

Say yes to yoga. Hunching over smartphones and tablets can lead to headaches and backache. Yoga eases the tension that hunching creates, clears the mind, and promotes positive thinking and problem-solving. A few simple sequences (sun salutation and downward dog) every day will loosen you up, strengthen core muscles and keep you flexible.

Meditate regularly. Take ten minutes every morning to meditate – sit quietly, read something inspiring or just think. Proven to combat depression, meditation can also reduce the risk of heart attack and stroke by up to 15 per cent.

Plan ahead. Healthy eating requires preparation. Most broken diets and cravings come from temptation, getting too hungry and not having healthy options to hand. Keep fresh fruit and vegetables in the fridge at home/work, and make up healthy batches of soup which can be frozen to eat throughout the week. Stock up on nutritious cupboard essentials (see Primal Eating) which make it easy to throw together a tasty meal in the evenings.

Ten-a-day. OK, the guidance says five-a-day, but you can manage more than that! Stick with seasonal fruit and vegetables, and make them a larger portion of every meal. Slice fruit onto your morning cereal or yogurt, and add a couple more veg to your salad at lunch or dinner.

Fifteen minutes of sun. Even if the sun isn't shining, get daylight on your skin for at least 15 minutes a day. Your body needs vitamin D to protect it from disease, including various cancers, and most of us are vitamin D deficient. Expose your arms and legs without sun protection, if possible (of course, though, safe sunscreen should be worn after 15 minutes, and in high temperatures). Being outside, even in weak winter sunlight, will also boost your mood and combat seasonal blues.

Get your omega-3s. Healthy fats are rich in omega-3s, and proven to lower cholesterol and strengthen the immune system. They also keep your joints, brain, heart and eyes (and so much more) in tip-top condition.

Berries and nuts. Go primal with your snacks! Blueberries are high in polyphenols, i.e. plant compounds that are powerful anti-inflammatories. They also improve blood flow and boost immunity. Cashew nuts, walnuts and almonds are packed with essential fats, protein and iron.

Prioritise sleep. Forget the Thatchers, Churchills and Wintours of the world, and make time for your Zzzs. Sleep-deprivation makes you less productive and more stressed; it can also make you look older and age faster. Getting more sleep improves everything.

From sunlight to snacks to sleep, these are just a few of the strategies you can use to boost your primal mindset. Many of these ideas are common sense, whereas others may be new to you. There are a lot of other key elements to reinforce your newfound positivity.

Pay close attention to how your mind is working. Listen to your inner voice, observe your reactions and watch how you interact with others. Negative thinking, rushing to judgement, assuming the worst and being overly critical are normal for the majority of us most of the time. Simply becoming aware of your automatic thoughts and self-talk can transform your mindset from habitually negative to typically positive.

As we've seen, gratitude can be immensely powerful. As you become more aware of the good in your life, other aspects of the primal mindset will follow naturally. Practising gratitude will help you to develop flexibility and resilience for when troubles or challenges arise in your life. You will also find it easier to avoid constant carping or criticism, so that you feel more naturally positive about yourself and others.

Adopting a primal mindset is about more than just positive thinking: it's a range of attitudes and perspectives which will make you a healthier person, both in body and soul. It will help you to work out what really matters and what doesn't, thus increasing your happiness and reducing stress. As you become more attuned to your gut instincts, you'll gain trust in your own feelings and learn to negotiate everyday decisions with ease.

Best of all, thinking primally will strengthen your inner confidence, making you more understanding of others, more forgiving of yourself and more thankful for the abundance of good in your life.

Chapter 2
Primal Disconnection

It is a truth universally acknowledged that time online passes at a different rate to time in the real world. When you're watching meerkats dancing on YouTube, hours can whizz by, whereas when you're sitting at work, waiting for the weekend, every minute seems to drag by... How does being connected to the great Internet god suck away so much of our precious time?

Constant digital connection has become the norm – and it's happened quite quickly. At the start of the twenty-first century we weren't all permanently online everywhere we went. In 2015 Facebook announced they had passed the landmark of over a billion users on a single day (Monday 24 August). That approximates to one in seven humans on the planet using Facebook. It's predicted that the number of smartphone users will exceed two billion in 2016.

These days it's normal to spend hours online, aimlessly surfing this virtual world, in the same way we spend hours watching TV or wandering around the shops buying 'stuff' we don't need. But do any of those activities make us any happier? A walk in the park or along the canal will refresh, recharge and restore you more than any website or window-shopping.

Time *is* precious. Let's not mince our words: old or young, sick or healthy, every human being on the planet is heading in the same direction. Time, for each and every one of us, is running out. Going primal, and therefore having made the decision to make each day just a little bit more meaningful, helps you to confront this fact. Disconnecting on a regular basis is essential to living more primally.

Try this simple exercise to kick-start your disconnection journey.

Disconnection Exercise

Find a cool, dark space where you can be alone and undisturbed. Lie down on a sofa, bed or the floor. Switch off your phone or disable all alerts.

Find a piece of music you find relaxing: it could be classical, ambient, choral or jazz. You could try 'The Lark Ascending' by Vaughan Williams, 'Kind of Blue' by Miles Davis, or anything by Massive Attack, Zero 7 or Portishead.

Close your eyes for the entire piece, inhaling and exhaling gently. Allow the music to permeate every inch of your body.

Visualise a calming scene, as the music builds and changes. Imagine green rolling hills or endless blues skies, an empty beach, crashing waves, or whatever else the music evokes for you.

Repeat this exercise every evening for a week. It won't take longer than ten or 15 minutes and is the perfect mental refresher.

Experiment with other tracks: make your own recharge-and-refresh playlist. You might try music you don't normally listen to, such as opera, electronic chill-out tracks or Gregorian chants.

Whatever you choose, make sure you're completely disconnected. For those ten or 15 minutes, it's just you, the music and the images in your head.

Monkey Brain

It's been estimated that the average human has 15,000–50,000 thoughts per day, most of which are repetitive and self-directed. In other words, we circle around the same thoughts or preoccupations with the same issues, so it's not surprising that we get stuck, feel frustrated and overheat sometimes. Harvard psychologists Matthew Killingsworth and Dan Gilbert estimate that for 47 per cent of the time, our mind is off wandering: 'Unlike other animals, humans spend a lot of time thinking about what is not going on around them; contemplating events that happened in the past, might happen in the future, or will never happen at all.'

Most of us will recognise this tendency to worry or obsess over the past and the future, to the extent that we miss out on the present. It's what meditation, mindfulness and brain training are all about: the attempt to stop what Buddhists call the constant 'monkey brain' and get control. Primal thinking helps to slow down our racing thoughts, and experience the here and now.

Primal Thinking

In a world which is becoming ever more virtual, digital and remote, going primal is a reassuringly human concept. Increasingly, our interactions with other human beings are not very human at all: we work 'remotely', and we demand faster Wi-Fi, sharper resolution and quicker connectivity. In all this hyper-activity, what we gain in speed, we lose in human connection.

Think back to – or imagine, if you can – the world before smartphones. How has your life/work changed? Are the changes generally positive or negative? And what about your daily routines? When was the last time you sat down and put pen to paper? When did you last write a postcard, thank-you note or even a shopping list? When did you last get talking to a random stranger in a café? When did you last eavesdrop on a conversation in a public place, just listening to people talking about something funny, sad or downright bizarre?

An activity as simple as chatting to the cashier in your local supermarket is lost when you pay at the electronic checkout. Enjoying the view as your train speeds through the countryside, catching sight of the first swallow of spring or glimpsing the face of a long-lost lover from the top deck of a London bus – we miss a lot when we're glued to our screens.

To Be or Not to Be

In summer 2015, the actor Benedict Cumberbatch made his much-anticipated debut as Hamlet at the Barbican. However, within a few nights of the first previews, the actor was begging his adoring fans to stop filming his performance. Addressing them outside the theatre, he said there was 'nothing less supportive' while on stage than seeing 'all these cameras, phones, filming me... I can see red lights in the auditorium. It's blindingly obvious... I want to give you a live performance that hopefully you will remember in your minds and brains, whether it's good, bad or indifferent, rather than on your phones, so please don't.' The *Hamlet* incident raised interesting questions about the live experience in the age of personal technology. We've all been in situations, such as at sporting events, in museums, galleries or tourist attractions, where visitors resemble a robotic barrage of mobiles, filming or snapping – but apparently not looking with their own eyes.

Whether it's filming that winning goal (and probably missing the action) or obstructing the view of others by holding a phone up during a concert, the way we experience live events is being transformed by technology. We have to work out how we feel about these issues. As human beings, we're relational, symbiotic, interdependent – whatever you want to call it, we gather in groups and share special events... But do we want to interact behind the barrier of our mini-screens?

What Have We Gained?

There is no doubt that technology has brought positive advances. There is more computing power, it is said, contained in a single smartphone than was used in NASA's first Moon landings in 1969. We have seemingly unlimited knowledge at our fingertips, and the ability to access it in seconds. The Internet is a leveller, a force for democracy and equality; we can study online, whether we live in Antarctica or Afghanistan, are rich or poor, young or old. We can interact with strangers about our passion for Norse mythology, raw-food cooking or street dance.

And then there's e-commerce: small businesses trading, selling and innovating with others all over the world. Online shopping is another positive development; forget lugging home heavy bags from the supermarket: now we can get those tins of baked beans and washing detergent delivered in bulk, at a time of our choosing. We can have work meetings via Skype and talk 'virtually' face to face with our loved ones across the world. Technology has cut down on flights, car journeys and pollution; it has boosted commerce and enterprise, and freed up time previously spent on shopping or commuting for more interesting pursuits. Only the most stubborn Luddite could deny that technology has changed many of our lives for the better.

However, the question remains: are we really connecting? The terminology of the digital revolution is all about 'connection' – it's said that the World Wide Web 'connects' you to the entire world. On one level this is accurate, as many have made lifelong friends or even met life partners online: it is a great way to forge new relationships. The Internet – with its countless special interest websites and discussion boards – has brought together many vulnerable or lonely people, bridging the geographical distance between us all.

On the other hand, there is also evidence that spending too much time in the virtual world can be profoundly isolating, damaging to human interaction and may even cause autistic-like social impairment. Scientific research shows that virtual contact with others cannot replace flesh-and-blood contact with other human beings: the cerebral cortex (the thinking part of the brain) registers digital contact, but the amygdala (the primitive part of the brain) does not. This explains why lack of human company makes us feel deprived and lonely.

Anxiety disorders (and associated conditions, such as depression and eating disorders) are thought to be increasing among the so-called Generation Y and Millennials. With more choices and more technology than ever before, they are struggling with information overload, constant comparison and a sense of failure. A 2014 American study found that female students spent an average of ten hours a day on their phones, and male students eight hours a day (Baylor University, Texas). Utah Valley University has installed separate lanes on campus, allowing students to 'walk', 'run' and 'text' (what happened to 'talk' or 'hold hands', you might ask).

Neuroscientist Baroness Susan Greenfield is well known for her controversial views on the damaging impact of technology on the human brain – especially those of children and young people. She has written about the risk of relying on screen dialogues (texting and emailing) to communicate, and wonders whether we will lose the ability to conduct real conversations in real time: 'Perhaps future generations will recoil... at the messiness, unpredictability and immediate personal involvement of a three-dimensional, real-time interaction.'

Greenfield is not the only one who believes that mass digitisation has a disproportionate and damaging effect on the young. As Steve Hilton argues in his book *More Human*: 'We are blasé about the impact of technology on children's lives, and at the same time are undermining one of the most natural, human... aspects of children's lives: play.' Like Greenfield, Hilton considers the all-pervasive obsession with online activity to be a threat to children's natural physical instincts to explore the world around them, to imagine and invent, and to play with others.

This digital overload starts early: many babies and toddlers are now completely at ease interacting with tablets and smartphones. According to the American Academy of Pediatrics, children spend an average of seven hours a day on entertainment media, online gaming and watching TV. According to a 2015 Ofcom report, 90 per cent of 16–24-year-olds own a smartphone.

Grown-ups are getting in on the act, too: Ofcom reported that 66 per cent of UK adults own a smartphone. Over-55s are also joining the revolution, with smartphone ownership among the 55–64 age group more than doubling since 2012, from 19 per cent to 50 per cent in 2015. Young and old, there's no doubt that we're increasingly hooked on our gadgets and enjoying being online. But where does this leave the more primal parts of our lives: our hearts and minds?

How to Unplug

For all the positive aspects of connection, we mustn't ignore the fact that people are also reporting more loneliness. It's as though we feel alone together: our smartphones and tablets offer an endless virtual world when what we actually need is real, human companionship. Adopting a more primal attitude to human connection simply means unplugging from technology once in a while.

You don't need to go back to a prehistoric, pre-industrial, pre-technological age, in order to stay sane. There are many easy, primal ways to find headspace among all the digital distractions. I have regular 'unplugged' weekends, with no email or Internet – a strategy I'd highly recommend. After a couple of days back in the real world, I always feel calmer and more connected to my partner, my friends and family. By Monday morning, my head is clearer, and I'm ready to tackle the working week.

A few years ago I was greatly influenced by something called the Sabbath Manifesto. Founded by a Jewish community group (but applicable to non-religious and religious alike) the manifesto encourages people to slow down their lives. They recommend regular disconnection from all forms of media and technologies.

The Sabbath Manifesto

Based on the traditional seventh day of rest, the ten core principles are as follows:

1. Avoid technology

2. Connect with loved ones

3. Nurture your health

4. Get outside

5. Avoid commerce

6. Light candles

7. Drink wine

8. Eat bread

9. Find silence

10. Give back.

It's not hard to see why these principles resonate with so many of us. They speak to a universal desire to return to a more natural way of being, in touch with our physical surroundings and our loved ones. They capture the essence of what a primal lifestyle looks like.

> **Pip, 43:** I bought an exercise bike last year and I was determined to get fit. I'm sitting down all day in the office, and it's far too easy to snack and not move around much at all. As a single mother I can't go out running or to the gym in the evenings – so I figured I could cycle a few miles a day, in front of the TV… Unfortunately, it hasn't worked out like that. I've used the bike about three times, and it's become that cliché, a clothes hanger. I have all the best intentions, but then I start fiddling around with my tablet and that's it – I've wasted an entire evening.

What Pip might need to do is to ban herself from going online for a fixed period of time – say half an hour – which she could devote to the exercise bike. As she points out, it's far too easy to get sucked into hours of empty Googling/tweeting/Instagramming/YouTubing.

This is not about being a digital refusenik: slowing down can co-exist alongside new technology. Tom Hodgkinson, founder of the Idler Academy, reflects on how digital technology can help the cause of slowness:

> *I've been through various rages about the internet. One, because it distracts from our idling time. And two, because it takes money away from traditional idling industries such as publishing and music. But I've calmed down about it now. People forget how intrusive the telephone used to be…*

Now, it hardly ever rings. It's much more civilised to check your emails at your leisure. And having a Blackberry means that I can genuinely sit in the pub and do my work. **"**
Evening Standard interview, 2015

Infomania

Would Einstein have come up with his theory of relativity if he'd focused on it for 30 seconds before moving on to checking his emails? Good work needs a primal mindset, a focused brain and deep, uninterrupted thought.

Humans are bombarded with around five times as much news, media and random Internet information than 30 years ago, on top of the thousands of pointless emails which make their way into our inbox every year. 'Brain-freeze' is an experience many of us are familiar with; also known as mind fog, it is a general feeling of being mentally scrambled, frazzled, burnt out. Technology enables us to switch between so many screens, apps and conversations at the same time that often we're not concentrating on any of them. Multitasking also increases the production of cortisol and adrenaline, which further over-stimulate the brain. What we call multitasking is often just switching rapidly between tasks, giving each one our fragmented attention and underperforming at them all. The brain is not wired to work this way.

Contrary to popular belief, doing several different things at once doesn't save time or increase efficiency. As well as making you feel rushed and stressed, it can impair cognitive performance.

According to the cognitive neuroscientist Dr Daniel Levitin, multitasking is a 'diabolical illusion' which results in confusion and disorganisation. Juggling too much different digital input causes the brain to miss out on the natural, daydreaming, resting state that it needs to function in everyday life. Every email, text or tweet we receive is effectively competing for mental space and attention – which leaves us less brainpower to think about the other important things in life, such as our finances, friends or family.

In his 2015 book, *The Organised Mind: Thinking Straight in the Age of Information Overload*, Levitin explains how trying to learn while multitasking actually misdirects the new information to the wrong part of the brain. Unread emails, tweets and TV stop information going into the hippocampus, the brain region where it can be organised and categorised, ready for retrieval.

Solo-tasking

Thinking primally not only helps to organise information in your brain more effectively, but it will also allow you focus on what really matters in your life. Whether it's an important work project, relationship troubles, a personal challenge, or even sleeping or eating problems, thinking primally can show you what you need to do and why. Disconnecting on a regular basis is an essential part of this process, helping to clear your head, and focus your mental efforts.

For many of us, concentration is becoming a dying art. While multitasking is necessary sometimes, it's also important to relearn how to focus. Levitin recommends ditching the gadgets and using old-fashioned pen and paper, because it forces our brains to process the information more deeply: 'The very act of writing something down causes you to remember it better...'

So, if you need to draft a difficult letter or a speech, or memorise something, use a pen and paper. Make notes, copy out information, get ideas down on the written page – it's a great way to work through it cognitively, discover links and fix it in your brain.

Another effective way to turn down the relentless mental chatter is to take time every day to solo-task. The more mundane the activity, the better: loading the dishwasher, feeding the cat, unloading the washing machine. Pull each damp item from the machine, inhale the freshness of the detergent and feel the texture of the material. If you're hanging it up to dry indoors, take time to arrange it on the clothes horse. More primal still, peg each item out on a washing line outdoors, pausing to feel the sun or breeze on your skin.

Focus on what you're doing and nothing else: there is plenty of time. Use each task, whether it's laundry, cat-feeding or even writing your shopping list, as a casual meditation. Check in with yourself.

Primal and Individual

At the heart of slowing down – and occasionally disconnecting completely – is individualism. This is often felt as a desire to work, eat and exist more meaningfully, to experience our lives as they pass, and to be who we really are.

As well as beginning to turn our backs on digital bombardment, we're increasingly sick of being told *how to be*. Modern life is liberal in many ways – freedom of religious expression or the greater acceptance of gender fluidity, for example – but curiously hectoring in others. The *shoulds* and *oughts* are usually directed at women, focusing especially around our personal lives and careers, what to eat, what to weigh, what to wear and how to look.

Deciding to live more primally removes you from this vortex of comparison, anxiety and judgement. Slowing down gives you time to look around and savour your food, your relationships and your world. It restores your confidence, and puts you back in touch with your body and in charge of your life.

Peak Selfie?

The average 16–25-year-old woman spends around five hours a week (or around 48 minutes a day) taking (and retaking and retaking) her selfies (according to research conducted by OnePoll in April 2015). Social media, reality TV, magazines and celebrity culture are all contributing to the rise in body dissatisfaction and depression among young people, and fuelling the rise in cosmetic procedures.

Have we reached peak selfie? The self-consciously posed 'duck face' selfie is starting to get tired. The tourists wielding selfie sticks which fill our towns and cities are beginning to become ridiculous. The writer Howard Jacobson describes the selfie stick as 'the lightning rod of narcissism'.

Social scientists have noted a correlation between the rise of the (selfish) selfie and a decline in altruism. When the camera was first invented, taking photographs was about looking outwards, capturing a beautiful view, iconic landmark or a gathering of loved ones. Now the camera is firmly trained on the taker, putting the individual at the centre of everything. Of course, there's a time and a place for including oneself in a scene – it's lovely to be able to join friends in a group photograph – but we should beware of the selfie-craze tipping into self-obsession.

Disconnect for Work

Disconnecting is good for your mental health, and it's also good for your work. In 2010 I attended a lecture given by the American novelist Jonathan Franzen. He said that he writes alone, in a bare office, wearing both earplugs and noise-cancelling headphones to block out the world. When writing his novel *The Corrections* (2001), he physically sealed up his Ethernet port to remove all possibility of connecting to the Internet.

Franzen calls himself a 'lifelong amateur', and is open about the failed novels and the 'pathetic' false starts. Each of his successful novels has taken him years to write, and it involved an epic struggle. The element of disconnection is central to this slow, agonising process; at that lecture he said something else which has stayed with me ever since:

> ❝ *It's doubtful that anyone with an Internet connection at his workplace is writing good fiction.* ❞

Franzen's point is clear, albeit deliberately provocative. The Internet sucks up our concentration, our mental juice and our productive time. Of course, it's also a fantastic tool, connecter of people and fount of all knowledge (and plenty of nonsense). But seeing how many amazing blogs, songs and products are out there can be weirdly discouraging, when you're trying to write or invent your own. Would Mozart have composed 'The Queen of the Night' aria in *The Magic Flute* if he had been online? (Go on, listen to it now and marvel!) Would Milton have written *Paradise Lost*? If you want to create, you should be doing just that, rather than aimlessly surfing around in cyberspace.

Ration Your Online Time

Of course, we need the Internet sometimes. Say, you're a writer like Franzen and you need to check something like a name, a place or a historical fact. Write yourself a list (with an actual pen and paper) and check facts online at the end of the day. The *end* of the day, not the beginning. I do this, adding to my checklist as I go, and it feels like a reward for a productive day's work.

Another writer, Joss Whedon, hit the headlines in 2015 when he decided to take some time off Twitter in order to reclaim his creativity: 'I just thought: "Wait a minute, if I'm going to start writing again, I have to go to the quiet place. And this is the least quiet place I've ever been in my life."'

Digital Addiction

There is no doubt that we're hooked on our screens: to be deprived of our phones – or to have no coverage – sends many of us into a panic. Up to 20 per cent of adults in the UK describe themselves as 'addicted' to their digital devices. When I worked in publishing, I remember that on the rare occasions when the network 'went down', we became utterly paralysed. We'd all sit there in front of blank screens, turning them off and on compulsively, ringing the IT helpdesk, unable to begin any useful work. Strange, isn't it? We had pens, notepads, functioning landlines and even our own brains, but we were rendered useless by the lack of working computers.

Many of our best intentions – getting fit, spending more time with the family, sorting out the garden or just getting more sleep – are derailed by the temptations of our gadgets. The constant distraction they provide is unlike anything humans have known before. Unlike going to the cinema, shopping or any other leisure activity which still requires a certain degree of patience, we don't need to wait: the online distractions contained within our phones are always on! You can watch, discuss, check or buy almost anything, anytime, right there on your screen. Wi-Fi is so widely available now that it can be difficult to disconnect even when you're actively trying to. Whenever I go into the British Library or a café to write, specifically switching off my phone to avoid distraction, my laptop detects the Wi-Fi and magically connects itself – and how tempting it is, a whole digital world out there just waiting to swallow me up.

This is a practical problem – we're surrounded by connectivity – but there are practical, positive, primal solutions to it.

Switching Off

- Disable notifications: receiving continuous alerts wreaks havoc with your concentration. You don't need to know every time an email arrives.

- Remove yourself physically from the tempting device: put your phone under a cushion in another room.

- Don't use your phone as an alarm – it's the first thing you see in the morning and before you know, you're online, checking emails, updating Twitter, and you've blown the morning inspiration.

- Don't go on social media first thing in the morning: your personal goals must come first (see below).

- Implement a tech-free mealtime rule: agree with your partner or other family members that you won't bring gadgets to the table. This frees you up to focus on good conversation and good food. Do the same when eating alone.

- Take it slow: if a detox day feels too much (or is impractical), start with a regular detox hour. Allocate just 60 minutes a day to unplugging and doing something REAL: take a bath, go for a run, walk your dog, bake a cake or listen to an entire album.

- Gradually, you can extend this detox hour to a detox day, or even a detox weekend (see the Sabbath Manifesto).

Occasionally, radical action is required. Once, faced with a looming deadline, I gave my phone to my best friend and made him promise not to give it back to me for a fortnight. It worked – even though I begged him to return it, he kept it, and I got the work done.

However, if you can be strict with yourself, there are ways to reclaim your own time.

- Decide on what you want to achieve: your personal goal.

- Your goal should be specific, measurable and achievable. For example, I will paint two walls in the bedroom, I will study Japanese for an hour after dinner, I will run twice around the block or I will weed the flowerbeds.

- Set a limit to how long you'll spend online in your free time, such as one hour in the evenings.

- Go online *after* the goal time: use it as a reward *when and only when* you have worked on the more important task, i.e. your goal.

Of course, if your work *is* the Internet – if you're a web designer, software engineer or the next Steve Jobs – you'll need to spend significant amounts of time in cyberspace, marketing, researching or programming your gizmos. Just as a violinist goes to concerts, or a vet spends time with animals, you'll need to be online. Similarly, freelancers need to be online, self-promoting and looking for new opportunities, as does anyone who works in a traditional 9–5 role.

Whatever your industry, though – whether you're freelance or a full-time employee – you still need to generate new ideas from your own brain. We could all benefit from time spent lying in a field, watching the flowers grow, or walking the city streets and observing our fellow human beings. Time away from the Internet is the ultimate opportunity for more positive, primal thinking and problem-solving.

Forget FOMO

Taking time 'off'-line can provoke anxiety: if you're not online, it sometimes feels like you're missing out. This really isn't the case. Everything will still be there when you log back on (in fact, everything will be there forever). You can banish FOMO (fear of missing out) by bearing in mind that you're not missing out on anything. In any case, is any of it as real as your real life? Social media creates a skewed version of human existence: the beautified, filtered version we choose to portray, in which our lovers send us flowers, the sun shines and our selfies come out perfectly. You're watching other people's highlight reel, not their real lives.

The writer Henry David Thoreau said: 'Most men lead lives of quiet desperation…' Depressing – but he has a point. Mostly life is taking out the bins and wondering what's that dry patch of skin behind your ear – not mini-breaks, fashion shows and cocktails with the girls. One of my friends tweeted a photo of herself in pristine workout gear looking ultra-fit at the gym and later told me: 'The funny thing is, I've only been twice since I joined!'

The Internet doesn't just portray an idealised version of our lives; it can also bring us down. Social media anxiety is a genuine problem: 45 per cent of young people said that social media leaves them feeling 'worried and uncomfortable'. Measuring your own happiness against the filter-fabulous profiles of other people (often strangers) can affect your mood, confidence and relationships.

The 'compare and despair' cycle of checking other people's profiles is pointless and self-defeating. Why compare their apparently perfect lives to your own, wondering why everyone else is living the dream while you're still at home with your parents? Why would we measure our own happiness against that of others, often people we don't even know? The most content people are not usually documenting every second of their lives on social media – they're out there actually living!

When the virtual world starts to have a negative impact on your life, or if it makes you feel inadequate in comparison with others, it's time to take action. Here are a few positive, primal strategies for regaining control of your digital habit.

Set limits: if you're spending all your time on social media, set yourself some boundaries. Maybe you'll check updates only twice a day or have weekends off.

Break the habit: try to break that automatic reflex of reaching for your phone when you're sitting on the bus/train, when waiting for a friend or when walking.

Open your eyes: spending less time on social media will give you more time in the real world! Notice the weather, look around you, and listen to the birds and the bees.

Clean up your settings: if specific profiles, feeds or 'friends' are getting you down, making you feel unhappy or anxious, be ruthless. Whether it's toxic school friends you haven't seen for years, exes or celebs, unfollow or mute them. This will help to clear out the negativity and comparison.

Make time for real friends: face to face! Meeting up for lunch or coffee is a rare treat these days – and will remind you how fantastic true friends are.

Do other things: don't forget that books, paintings and films exist too. Turn off your phone and watch a DVD, or make a start on that book you've been wanting to read.

Remember: the Internet will still be there when you get back to it, with its cats and dogs juggling tennis balls and other people's superfood green smoothies. The difference is that you'll have started achieving something far more important: your personal goal. When you're working towards your own success, you'll find you care less about what other people are up to.

Quick Tip to Get Some Headspace...

Get a phone cover! It's simple and it really works. If you get a wallet-style model, it flips over, covers the light and stops the constant distraction. You know that thing, when you're reading a book or a magazine, and the phone starts flashing beside you? How long do you wait to check it – two seconds? Five seconds? A flashing message indicator is almost impossible to ignore. I bought a nice old leather cover for my smartphone, and it has really helped.

One of the simplest ways to disconnect, in six words:
Take a walk. Without your phone.

Curb Your Ego

In my circle, social media usage falls into three broad camps: food, fashion and politics.

- The first group are endlessly sharing images of what they've baked, what their partner cooked them for dinner and how beautiful their salad looks. This group includes 'tweet-before-you-eat' pics of their plates in restaurants and virtuous post-workout green juices.

- The second group share expert selfies of their super-stylish outfits, their vintage finds, quirky headwear, and coloured tights and amazing shoes. They also like to show off their latest hair and make-up looks. How do they start the day looking so *soigné*?

- The third group are constantly opining on current affairs: from who should win the election to why we should be spending more/less on international aid, and why politicians are hypocritical or have Got It Wrong. They also offer strong thoughts on celebrity matters. (This third group includes me.)

These are my broad social media groups of friends – even though, on reflection, I don't have that much in common with them. Your groups might include funny tweeters, sporting inspirations, Members of Parliament or just people who post images of cute kittens. Have you ever wondered why you're actually following them?

Our own social media contributions can be just as random. Why do you feel the need to show your breakfast to your Instafans or express your public outrage at the fact that your train is delayed? I often ask myself this question. Until the early twenty-first century, this continuous running commentary on the most mundane thoughts passing through our heads was not needed, desirable or even possible.

Here's a fantastic corrective to this kind of mindless drivel: **no one actually cares**. Harsh but true! No one needs your (my) minute-by-minute analysis of what is happening in the world. Stream of consciousness is all well and good, but keep it zipped up (or write it down).

Oversharing is not just tedious, but it can also make life a bit... cheap. We devalue our own thoughts, opinions and experiences by constantly feeling the need to air them, and get feedback or approval from others.

The psychiatrist and business consultant Leandro Herrero argues that we're rapidly becoming a 'full-disclosure society', egotistically addicted to clicks, likes and retweets. He believes that it's only by facing up to our egos, and realising that no one cares about what we think, that we can wean ourselves off oversharing.

Herrero has formulated the 'Border Diet': ten rules for reclaiming your personal borders.

1. Make a list of secrets.

2. Take a social-media sabbatical for a weekend.

3. Have moments alone, not doing anything.

4. Recognise your assets and strengths – and don't give them away for free.

5. Practise silence.

6. Practise stillness.

7. Avoid mental pollution. Don't go to a chat room full of trivia: it's bad for your soul.

8. Don't be fooled by your ego – the world does not care.

9. It's OK to have borders. Protect them and know what is sacred and secret.

10. Go back to number one.

These are funny and relatable suggestions (especially number 8). It's not only 'OK' to have borders – it's essential. Just as tweeting about your private life cheapens those intimate moments (do you really need to live-tweet your marriage proposal or giving birth?), so sharing every random event devalues your existence. Any one of us who uses social media could benefit from retreating a little into our own lives, quieting down the 'clever dick' comments. When you find silence in your own head, you feel more content in your own life.

Primal Reconnection

It may well cheapen our private experiences, but perhaps there's another reason for our tendency to overshare. While digital communication is weirdly impersonal, it's also driven by that most primal of all desires: human interaction and community. It's a sort of existential cry in the dark, seeking self-affirmation or reassurance. The more remote our lives become, the more we need to make these connections. I don't believe that it's all humblebragging and over-opinionated narcissism. In fact, when we share our thoughts on the Eurovision song contest, or post comments on any collective events, we're not just saying: 'Do you think this, too?' Ultimately, we're asking that deeply human question: 'Is there anybody out there?'

For all the benefits of technology and all the positive reaching out and sharing we do online, we need to stay connected to what's real. Disconnecting regularly, however briefly, is like closing the door on the outside world when it gets too noisy and hectic. It's a great way to reconnect with the important people and relationships in your life, and with your natural surroundings. Disconnecting from the virtual world helps you to get perspective in troubled times: a long walk can sort out emotions in a way that the Internet can't. Disconnecting reminds your primal brain how to think for itself, without a million Wikipedia pages or other people's opinions crowding in. Disconnecting will help you to sleep more deeply, think more clearly and experience life more intensely.

Chapter 3

Primal Relationships

In January 2006, the body of a woman named Joyce Vincent was discovered in a North London flat. She had been dead since approximately December 2003. She was 38 years old. Her body, so decomposed as to be barely identifiable, was lying surrounded by Christmas presents that she had wrapped but not delivered. Her heating and electricity were still running, covered by direct debits, and the television had been on continuously since her death. Neighbours had attributed the smell of decomposing body tissue to the downstairs bins.

Vincent's unnoticed death is sad beyond words, but it's also alarming. How could it happen? How did we get to a stage where a young woman could simply disappear without anyone telephoning or popping round, wondering about her whereabouts or caring... Vincent was not some social outcast, felled by addictions or homelessness. After her death people remembered her as beautiful, intelligent and successful. She is thought to have had a fiancé, she had previously worked at a global accountancy firm and she came from a 'nice family'. How could neighbours, colleagues or friends not have looked for her while she lay there dead for nearly three years?

(If you're interested to know more, Carol Morley's moving film 'Dreams of a Life' tells the whole story.)

Only Connect
At the heart of primal relationships is that simple concept: connection.

The UK was recently voted the loneliness capital of Europe. We're less likely to have strong friendships we can rely on and less likely to know our neighbours than most of our European counterparts. One in ten Brits does not feel they have even one close friend. According to Age UK, more than a million older people have not spoken to another person in the past month.

We're always hearing that new technology is bringing people closer than ever before, but many still feel isolated. For all the high-speed broadband in the world, levels of loneliness and depression are on the increase. Suicide remains the leading cause of death among British men under 50 years of age: more than a quarter of men who die between the ages of 20 and 34 take their own lives, and 13 per cent of deaths among men aged 35–49 are self-inflicted. (The figures for British women in the same age brackets are 13 per cent and five per cent, respectively.)

What does it mean to connect with others? Skype and Facetime enable you to see the face of the person you're talking to, but the experience is still pretty disembodied. At every important occasion, from birthdays, weddings or a child's first nativity play to a global summit, humans gather together. We pay large sums of money to attend live sports events, music concerts or theatre performances. Sure, we can use Skype and video-conferencing for work, but it's no substitute for a face-to-face meeting. We could watch those live events online, but we prefer to be there with others, listening to the real thing. The virtual experience just isn't the same.

Primal Ways to Beat Loneliness

Be brave: don't wait to be asked – get involved! Whether it's a work, social or school event, don't lurk on the sidelines. Shyness can be mistaken for standoffishness; after all, no one will know you want to take part unless you speak up. Volunteer to help organise the office party, the school fete or a book group: this is the best way to start conversations and, hopefully, friendships.

Be honest: if you feel lonely but are forever putting on a 'front', giving the impression that you're wildly busy and successful, don't be surprised when people assume you are! We often use social media to portray these fictional happy lives, so people think we're doing fine. There is no need to broadcast your loneliness to the whole world, but try being honest with those you trust – you'll be surprised how many others feel the same way.

> Let go of perfect: be realistic about your standards for yourself and others. There is no such thing as a perfect friendship: most friends let you down occasionally, just as you let them down. Ask yourself, would you prefer to be alone or have fun with others, warts and all? Being great mates is good enough!

> Step away from the computer/TV: increasingly, our virtual online worlds, TV and box sets give us the impression of being with others when we're actually alone. There's a time and place for cosy nights in and great 'virtual' buddies, but there's also a time and place for real human company. Switching off the gadgets and getting out there will force you to be sociable, meet others and make new friends. Regular social contact is essential for our primal health and well-being.

> Join a meet-up: if your social circle still feels small, find a group of like-minded people online. Thousands of people every year make contact on the web and meet up face to face, through anything from reading or gardening or coding clubs, to local mum-and-baby groups, to special interest societies.

However lonely you feel, you're not alone. Being brave, being honest and being out there are the first steps to forging some real human connections. Deep down we know that nothing replaces flesh-and-blood conversation, physical company and human intimacy. As Aristotle wrote, c.335 BC, 'Man is by nature a social animal.' People need to be around people, to be close to and talk to and touch – not just texts and likes and emoji hugs.

Friendship

Aristotle considered *philia* – translated as friendship, brotherly feeling, affection – as the highest form of love. And yet friendship is often taken for granted. We get caught up in partner relationships, the ups (and downs) of dating, hook-ups, falling in and out of love, marriages and divorces. In all that romance, turbulence and drama, it's easy to forget about friends; those steadfast pals who are there through thick and thin. We should value and nurture the friendships in our lives, because they're there for us when other things fall apart.

Primal friendship means caring about someone else's happiness or hurt. It's taking someone else as seriously as you take yourself: their safety, their sadness, their hopes, their triumphs and struggles. As we're not genetically related to these friends (and so have no evolutionary interest in their survival), you could say that Aristotle's *philia*, or friendship love, is the closest we get to true selflessness.

Friends – the real kind, not the Facebook kind – also fight each other's corner. This is important, especially when you're being a bit irrational or unreasonable. When others encourage you to see the other side of the argument, a best friend takes your side against all others. *Of course, it's outrageous your boss is treating you like that! As for that guy who hasn't texted you back? His loss!* Close friends listen and sympathise with these rants, and then they help to calm you down, control your emotions and find a solution.

Remember the Gore Vidal comment: 'Every time a friend succeeds something inside me dies.' We can all identify with that secret *Schadenfreude*, where the success of another feels like a personal defeat. However, in the most primal friendships, this secret competitiveness is absent: you rejoice in your friend's victory as if it were your own. The stronger and more secure you are in yourself, the more you can support your friends.

I had a boss who used to say: 'Strong people stand up for themselves, but stronger people stand up for others.' We should all champion our friends like this.

Primal Happiness

Connecting with friends makes us happy. Speaking at the Hay Festival in 2015, Professor Paul Dolan identified five ways we can all be immediately happier:

1. Listen to a favourite piece of music

2. Spend five more minutes with someone you like

3. Go outdoors

4. Help someone else

5. Have a new experience.

What could be more primal? Spending time with friends, being outdoors and helping others are all about connecting. As humans, this is the most primal thing we do.

Dolan, a professor at the London School of Economics, believes that many of the things people believe will make them happy are fleeting and can actually alter their lives in a negative way. 'Most things we think will make us happy won't. We're really always happier if we are focusing on the person we are with and the thing we are doing right now.'

Happiness, on a primal level, is a surprisingly simple equation: it's made up of the things we're doing and the people we're with, right now. Untold riches don't appear to make us happier: numerous studies have shown that earning *more* money doesn't increase personal happiness. Of course, up to a certain level, material wealth contributes to mental and physical ease and comfort, but beyond a certain level – usually set at around £50,000 – people do not appear to keep getting happier. Career success or greater power at work isn't the answer either: getting a promotion is likely to lead to longer working hours and more stress. Something as primal as spending time with friends, on the other hand, really can increase our levels of happiness.

The HBO series *Girls,* and *Friends* and *Sex and the City* before it, have found global popularity with their portrayal of these amazingly close groups of women. But how many of us really hang out with our bosom buddies like that? I see my hairdresser more often than I see some of my best friends, and I'm not the only one. While I love the technology that keeps us so close – we share *everything* over text or email – ringing or actually meeting up can seem somehow complicated.

Phone-phobic?

Text messages have long surpassed telephone calls as the preferred means of communication. Three years ago, 96 per cent of smartphone users spoke on their device at least once a week; now that number is more like 75 per cent. According to research (carried out by Ipsos MORI for Deloitte, September 2015) the amount of time a typical UK smartphone user spends on non-voice activities has almost trebled since 2012 to reach 90 minutes a day. Along with texts, instant messaging services, such as WhatsApp, iMessage and Snapchat, have become hugely popular: it's estimated that over 30 billion WhatsApp messages are sent every day, globally.

Many developmental psychologists warn that a generation are growing up without the art of conversation. Acronyms and emojis are inventive and expressive in their own way, of course, but they leave out an entire dimension of interpersonal skills which real-life interaction demands.

According to the media regulator Ofcom, around 93 per cent of UK adults now own a mobile phone, 80 per cent have broadband and 72 per cent use social networking sites. Technology is changing the way we relate to and communicate with each other. For all the connecting we're busily doing on our phones, this is mostly just virtual. Engagements and new babies are acknowledged with a brief tweet, a like or favourite.

Communication itself can be tricky: how often do you pick up the phone these days or drop round to see people unannounced? I rarely do. There's no doubt that we still want to communicate, but we prefer it to be indirect. A friend recently commented, 'I find unscheduled calls intrusive... like, why would you just call out of the blue? What if I'm doing something – can't you just email instead so I can deal with it in my own time, instead of invading my private space? If I'm calling a friend I have to psych myself up first.'

I know how she feels. But why, considering that we've grown up with the telephone, should making a call provoke anxiety? Is it the awkwardness and improvisation involved? Sending texts or emails is controllable, whereas real-time phone calls put you on the spot. There is the real risk of being caught off-guard: invited to something or asked directly to do something you don't want to do. Making excuses is far easier by text or email.

Then there's the awkwardness of speaking and overlapping, interrupting and clashing – *no you go first, sorry, haha! No it's fine, after you.* Not to mention the dreaded how-to-say-goodbye ritual. Have you ever hung up after several minutes of drawn-out, super-cheery *we-must-meet-up-really-soon* awkward farewells and cringed at your complete inability to do something as simple as terminate a phone call?

A survey by Deloitte predicts that the number of people who never make actual calls on their smartphone will rise to a quarter by the end of 2016, and that there will be virtually no smartphone users left *talking* by 2020. That may seem far-fetched, but there's no doubt of the extent to which speech has been usurped by other forms of communication. We're rapidly becoming conversation-avoidant, if not downright conversation-phobic.

As we dodge phone calls, we're turning into a world of textroverts – defined by the Urban Dictionary as: a) one who feels an increased sense of bravery over texting, as opposed to in person, and b) one who will often only say what they really feel over text messages.

Interaction feels easier when you are behind a screen. If things get tricky, you can just log off, divert the call, block the tweeter or delete the texts. But real-life meetings and direct conversations are important. Without them, we can't practise how to communicate with others, deal with uncomfortable situations and interpret non-verbal cues, such as visual cues and body language. Without the latter, we lose the ability to function in different social contexts and to work out how to flirt, apologise or console. The US psychologist Sherry Turkle is one of the leading researchers looking into the effects of technology on interpersonal development. Too much texting, she warns, amounts to a life of 'hiding in plain sight'.

Without real-life communication, we also lose a special dimension of what it means to be really, primally human.

Primal Pals

With all this call-dodging and indirect chat, how are we to reconnect with each other? What does primal friendship look like? Perhaps it starts with seeing each other more. Few of us would dream of having a relationship where we never saw our partner. And the same goes for friends. Whether it's a coffee once a week, dinner once a month or even a weekend visit once a year, face-to-face meetings remind you why you became friends in the first place.

Primal Friendship

Ring a good friend you haven't seen for a while and suggest meeting up for a coffee, a drink or a bite to eat. Just pick up the phone impromptu and do it! If you're both busy with childcare or work commitments, find creative solutions – meet each other on your lunch break, take children/dogs to the playground or do your supermarket shop together. Sometimes when I see my sisters, one of us will be doing household chores while we chat but it doesn't detract from the enjoyment of meeting up. You can even do an exercise class together before work. It really *is* different, seeing the people you love in real life.

Primal Kindness

Another primal ingredient for strong relationships is putting others first. Being kind is an underrated quality. Happy people are usually unselfish: selflessness seems to bring its own rewards. Best of all, they genuinely enjoy their lives. Everyone benefits when we all think collectively about the group, the family and the community. This doesn't mean being a doormat; it simply shows that you strive to think and act beyond your own interests, preferences and ego.

Joanna Lumley has a lovely take on everyday kindness: 'Every day I try to make life better for someone. It could be picking up a piece of paper. Being kind to someone or helping someone, sending off a small cheque for £10.'

Cheerfulness is another underrated quality. When life gets grim, when the news is full of human misery, spreading happiness really makes a difference. Just like smiling can trick your body into feeling happier, helping others is an instant way to improve your mood. If you can't make life better for yourself, why not make it better for someone else?

Niceness, or kindness – whatever we call it – is also deeply primal. If human beings hadn't co-operated with each other for thousands of years – those early primal gestures such as taking in an orphaned child when their parents were slain by wild boar or sharing food around the campfire – we would never have survived. Community is based on acts of kindness, ranging from the heroic to the mundane: it could be as simple as babysitting for a friend who needs a night off or just offering to get someone's lunch when you're going to the supermarket.

❝ *Practice random acts of kindness and senseless acts of beauty.* **❞**
US bumper sticker

It's easy to despair of our increasingly selfish, materialistic and atomised society – but maybe we're not that bad after all. At times, communities of strangers come together in surprising ways. In early 2015 in a suburb of Gateshead, a disabled pensioner called Alan Barnes was mugged while taking his bins outside. Only 4'6", and visually impaired, he was knocked to the ground and had his collarbone broken. A young beautician called Katie Cutler launched an online appeal with the aim of raising around £500 to help him get back on his feet. In the end, nearly 25,000 strangers donated, raising over £330,000.

Eventually it was Barnes, overwhelmed by the amount of money strangers had pledged, who asked for the fundraising to be halted. Katie Cutler was a stranger, too: she didn't know Alan Barnes, but she heard what happened to him and was moved by it. Some news stories just stop you in your tracks.

The photographer Jenny Lewis has spent the past five years documenting the experiences of new mothers and their babies in the first 24 hours after birth. Lewis's book, *One Day Young*, includes some moving example of kindness.

One of the women she photographed was a single mother. This mother had met an elderly woman at a bus stop a week before having her baby. The elderly woman, a complete stranger, insisted that the expectant mother move into her spare bedroom before the baby was born so that they wouldn't be alone – and that's where she and her new son were photographed, a few hours after his birth.

Lewis reflects on this simple act of kindness: 'What if everyone did something? If you cooked dinner for somebody because you knew they were on their own, or you offered to take their five-year-old to the playground to give the woman time for a shower?' Think how much these gestures would mean to you, coming from someone else. The smallest actions can sometimes have the biggest impact. We could all make time for a bit more altruism in our lives.

Get Involved

Taking part – whether it's local politics, team sports or your neighbourhood street party – is good for your health. Research consistently indicates that people with strong social networks live longer, healthier and happier lives. Getting involved is positive and primal; it's about being present in your physical environment, where you actually live, instead of virtually interacting in cyberspace.

In Primal Mindset we looked at the importance of learning to say no, whether to work or other obligations. But this is different: don't say no when it's something you want to do. Say yes if it's fun or a bit insane, such as climbing a mountain with your best friend or learning to skydive. Say yes when something inside you screams: 'Wow, if only I had the courage to do that!' Say yes when someone weaker or worse off needs your help. Say yes even when you're not sure you have the time. As the saying goes: *commit. You'll figure it out.*

Getting involved isn't all about fun. Increasingly, people are showing their support for serious causes around the world. After decades of individualistic capitalism, we're seeing a shift towards community, and collectivism, especially among the young. Witness the resurgence in grass-roots movements, localism and political activism. From the unprecedented Scottish National Party support at the Independence

Referendum in late 2014, to the tidal wave of anti-austerity politics sweeping Europe, from Podemos in Spain to Syriza in Greece, to the election of the ultra-left-wing MP Jeremy Corbyn as leader of the UK Labour Party.

The crisis across the Middle East has had tragic consequences, leading to the suffering and death of thousands of refugees trying to reach Europe – but there is also cause for optimism. There has been an outpouring of kindness, solidarity and compassion among millions of European citizens determined to show a welcome to their fellow human beings, whether from Syria, Iraq or Afghanistan. This is primal humanity in action.

Shared Living

Perhaps the reason we find kindness so rare, and yet so powerful, is that most of us live in carefully created private households: an intimate twosome, a family of four, a close-knit group of friends and housemates. It can be hard to let others into these private worlds or to consider sharing and living more closely with others. Do you know the names of your neighbours? Do you take in parcels for each other, pop in to feed the cat while they're on holiday or invite each other in for a cuppa? How would you feel about living alongside others?

While it's commonly thought that communal living ended with the hippie era of the 1960s, shared housing may be on the way back. Intentional communities – defined as people who live together on the basis of explicit common values – are seeing something of a resurgence. With the housing crisis and rising costs, the co-operative or co-housing movement makes financial sense too. Rising divorce rates have also contributed to this trend, as has the decline in multigenerational living. As early as 2010, the *Telegraph* reported on the rise of 'middle class communes' and mortgage companies have seen an increase in enquiries for co-housing financing.

Co-operative housing, where neighbours share services, skills and possessions, is a return to the way human beings used to live: from early primal communities in caves to more recent close-knit communities in small villages. Throughout most of the twentieth century, families shared ovens for baking bread and mangles for laundry, and children played outside in public green spaces. And it could be a solution to our dysfunctional, overpriced housing market: in 2011, 4.5 million people were on social housing waiting lists in England, and private-sector rents have increased by around 20 per cent in the last five years. The proportion of people owning their own homes, meanwhile, is expected to fall from a high of 72.5 per cent in 2001 to 63.8 per cent in 2021.

Shared housing communities range from self-defined, intentional, rural communes committed to sustainable living and a low-carbon lifestyle to looser communities in which shared cooking and cleaning rotas are the extent of their communal living. Neighbours, or co-habbers, share precious resources, such as washing machines, heating systems, lawnmowers and other tools (after all, why do we all buy this expensive machinery?!). Communities have laundry rooms and allotments; many have work co-ops, rotating gardening, painting and other general maintenance. Some have shared guest quarters for when relatives come to stay, and others even have communal pianos.

Sometimes they gather together like-minded artists, musicians and creatives, but not always. Communal living also works for young professionals unable to get on the housing ladder or older singletons, affluent and independent, who simply enjoy the company of others. Communal living may at last be losing those connotations of a hippy 'squat'.

Sharing chores and childcare, raising chickens and distributing the eggs, is part of a new green paradigm. With an overpopulated planet, many co-habbers see this as a practical way to reduce their environmental footprint. We have grown used to private units of a single person, couple or individual families, but it doesn't have to be that way. Whether it's as a result of baby boomers who are sick of their capitalist, individualistic lifestyles, or single or older people looking for company, or simply an awareness of the environment's dwindling resources, communal living could be the future.

This communal pulling together solves many of the problems of modern life. Younger residents can take on strenuous domestic chores, while older or frail ones might cook or look after children – it makes total sense. Not only is this a solution to the costs of childcare, it also helps with the growing problem of older people living longer, often alone, and sometimes in poor health. Insularity, or personal 'defensible space', does not have to be the norm. Living alone – dying alone – is not the only way. Socially, financially and environmentally, these friendly, flexible eco-communities make perfect, primal sense.

Primal Dating

Tinder, Grindr and OKCupid might not be particularly primal, but wanting to be close to other human beings is.

Tinder was only invented in 2012 and already has over 91 million users worldwide. Apps like that have been blamed for creating a consumerist attitude to relationships: a dehumanising process of judging or rejecting others solely on the basis of their photograph. The selection does appear somewhat brutal: swipe right if you fancy someone and swipe left if you don't. Not only does this remove subtlety and personality from the dating process, it cuts out the human dimension: all those indefinable aspects which make up interpersonal attraction. Few of us would choose our life partners based on a single photo: instead we're attracted to their voice, their smell, their presence, their kindness, their intelligence and the way they are.

Online dating has also been blamed for fuelling the 'grass is always greener' mindset. If a relationship hits a sticky patch and your girlfriend or boyfriend is annoying you, instead of persevering or learning to compromise, why not just look online and replace them with someone better? With thousands of potential partners at your fingertips, it's tempting to feel that you can simply upgrade.

> **Colin:** I first joined a dating website around five years ago, and I've been using apps for the last year. I had a few relationships at the start, but now I hardly ever go on dates: Tinder has become more of a habit than a way to meet anyone. At the beginning I put a lot

of time into looking at photographs, reading women's profiles, trying to find a good match. I used to feel hurt if they didn't reply to my messages or swipe me back. Now it's just water off a duck's back – when you get rejected ten or 20 times a day, you stop caring. I'd still like an actual girlfriend but to be honest I doubt if I'll meet her online.

When it comes to choice, less is sometimes more. Human beings may think we want a limitless selection, but when we get it, we're not very good with it. The American psychologist Barry Schwartz, author of *The Paradox of Choice*, has argued that unlimited choice can be a source of extreme anxiety for consumers. He believes that the proliferation of options, far from being liberating, is in fact debilitating, arguing that 'choice, and with it freedom, autonomy, and self-determination, can become excessive, and that when that happens, freedom can be experienced as a kind of misery-inducing tyranny. Unconstrained freedom leads to paralysis'.

Schwartz cites the experience of going shopping and being confronted with 285 different brands of cookies, 230 soups, 275 varieties of cereal, over 300 shampoos, and so on. The average American supermarket now carries nearly 50,000 items, more than five times what was available in 1975. Our primal brains have evolved, sure, but not to deal with this kind of commercial overload.

The psychologists Iyengar and Lepper designed an experiment to examine the effects of all this choice on human happiness. They randomly placed individuals in either a group where they could choose from 30 types of chocolate or a group in which they could choose from six types of chocolate. While subjects initially reported liking having the choice of 30 chocolates, they ended up being more dissatisfied and regretful of the choices they made than those who only had the choice of six. Not only do we find it harder to make decisions, but we're also less satisfied overall with the decision we make. We worry that we might have made the wrong one.

The more chocolates (or potential partners) you have, the harder it is to make a commitment. And we all know that attraction depends on more than just a pretty photo and a few pithy words.

Primal Instinct

The Internet has put power and information firmly in the hands of the consumer. We can research everything, from our choice of hotel for a weekend break to our medical treatment and our doctor's previous performance, in exhaustive detail before making decisions. Taking the same attitude to meeting a real-life partner, however, doesn't always work.

Dating apps and websites have their strengths, and can be a great way to make contact with like-minded souls. They offer a far greater pool of potential partners than you would normally meet in daily life. However, virtual attraction is not reality. If you're serious about having an actual relationship, it's important to meet up as soon as possible 'In Real Life'. On-screen you can become very close very quickly, writing and flirting, bonding and building up false expectations. (In research, older online daters tended to wait longer before meeting IRL, and were disappointed with the reality.) Physical human attraction is where our primal instincts and intuition really kick in.

You should also be clear about what you want. Some websites have been accused of promoting a 'hook-up' culture – people more interested in sex than long-term relationships. This may be true, but it's not necessarily a bad thing. A friend of mine uses Tinder in precisely this way: she is single, works long hours and enjoys having no-strings-attached sex. If that's the case, and you're taking care of your safety, that's fine. But if you're actually looking for a partner, perhaps to marry or start a family, you may be better off using traditional websites. There is nothing wrong with being honest about what you're looking for.

When you first meet someone, primal instincts are everything. In the words of the mighty Taylor Swift, 'I knew you were trouble…' Remember why the human gut has been called the second brain, and trust your intuition. Smell, for example – with the power of pheromones, your body will quickly tell you if you're drawn to another person. If your body is telling you that someone isn't right for you, listen. If a situation feels threatening or unpleasant, make your excuses and leave. If someone strikes you as too good to be true, a smoothie or a player, they probably are. As well as those primal instincts, remember to be safe: arrange to meet in a public place, and always tell a friend where you're going and when you'll be back.

He's Just Not That Into You...

... is the title of the best-selling book (2004), later a film (2009) and possibly the wisest phrase in the history of relationship advice. The message is beautifully straightforward and primal: if the person you're dating doesn't seem to be completely into you then they're probably not. We've all wasted time trying to decode the dreaded 'mixed messages' in new relationships, when actually they're not mixed at all. How do you act when you really like someone? Keen, right? How should someone act when they really like you? Keen, too.

When dating, tune into the primal messages your body is sending: your brain, your heart and your gut. If someone doesn't appear that keen on you, or isn't treating you well, be honest with yourself: if they're not making the effort to see you, it's probably because they don't want to.

Of course, in a long-term relationship there may be all sorts of reasons why someone appears withdrawn or preoccupied – and you should talk to them about it. But if you've only just started dating and someone is sending out mixed messages, don't waste your time.

You may think this sounds old-fashioned, even sexist or unfeminist: men doing the chasing and women waiting around for them to call? Not at all: it's as relevant to same-sex relationships as it is to heterosexual ones. Nothing is more demeaning than allowing someone to treat you badly, which includes not returning your calls, repeatedly leaving you hanging, cancelling dates and generally not making you feel amazing.

It's logical, when you stop to think about it, and liberating too. This rule is simple: don't pursue people who aren't interested and don't allow anyone to treat you badly. Adopting a zero-tolerance attitude to game-playing puts you back in control, and will bolster your confidence and self-respect. When you're not waiting around for someone who isn't interested, you're free for the next person who comes along and finds you irresistibly sexy.

Primal Sexiness

One of my favourite blogs is Marc and Angel Hack Life. A real-life couple and professional coaches, they're full of ideas for positive living. Their blog entitled '7 sexy character traits of happy people' argues that real sexiness is much subtler and more complex than physical appearance, body shape or wardrobe. In our over-sexualised society, overt raunchiness and exposed flesh have lost their allure, along with pouty selfies, endless over-sharing and sex tapes. Sexiness comes from your heart, mind and soul, joy and passion, a state of being.

Like me, Marc and Angel believe that sexiness is a mindset rather than a set of physical attributes. Here, slightly adapted from their blog, are a few of the sexiest character traits.

1. Consistent self-responsibility: happy people accept responsibility for how their life unfolds. They believe that their own happiness is a result of their thinking, beliefs, character and behaviour. The opposite is a whining, snivelling, accusing, blaming, irresponsible victim of life... NOT SEXY!

2. True (and humble) self-confidence: happiness requires a degree of confidence that allows us to believe we have value, and are worthy of love, friendship and success. Genuine self-love, as displayed by someone who feels comfortable in their own skin, is sexy and attracts others – cocky, shouty, boasty pseudo-confidence is not.

3. Self-acceptance: happy people are authentic. They are real, and know who they are and what they like. They spend time learning, growing and developing. They forgive their own shortcomings, but don't excuse them and instead work to transform themselves.

These character traits are definitely sexy and also deeply primal. They're about genuine self-love and honesty – about learning to value and cherish yourself – and the very opposite of pretence, self-deceit, avoidance, blame or bitterness. They're about accepting yourself as you are, while still striving to be better. This kind of inner calm, self-awareness and forward momentum are at the heart of a positive, primal mindset – and that will always be sexy.

Building Healthy Relationships

Online dating is one thing, but settling into a long-term relationship is quite another. Showing compassion to strangers is one thing, but our personal relationships are quite another! In some ways the relationships with those we don't know are more straightforward than relationships with those we do. Giving money to charity or donating unwanted possessions can often be far easier than dealing with the foibles and quirks of our nearest and dearest.

From rage to desire, irritation to affection, it's common to feel many different emotions for our loved ones in a single day, sometimes all at the same time. We want to protect them and simultaneously scream at them; be close to them and also have our own space. There's no doubt that our most intimate, romantic relationships can also be the most problematic. Here are some primal principles to bear in mind.

Nobody's perfect. Your partner isn't perfect, but neither are you. Often these quirks are what sparked the attraction in the first place. Maybe they're messy, or forgetful, but incredibly tolerant. Maybe they take ages getting ready to leave the house (mine does) but this same patience and slowness is a wonderful gift when they're listening to your problems. Bad sides have good sides. Don't expect them to be perfect, as no one is. Find someone whose imperfections can fit your own.

Learn to forgive. We all make mistakes – sometimes big ones. Being able to forgive is good for you as well as for others. The inability to forgive holds you back.

Learn to say sorry. This is part of growing up, like paying rent and taking the bins out! You are not always right. And even if you are, sometimes it's better to be happy than to be right.

Get over it. Resentment builds and festers. Don't be one of those bitter people who hold on to grudges from events in the distant past. Don't let feuds with family or friends drag on for years: be the bigger person and make amends. On a smaller scale, with a partner, don't let the sun go down on an argument: try to kiss and make up before bed.

The Big J. Jealousy is a big problem in any relationship. It's a very human emotion, but also extremely destructive and manipulative, and good relationships can be destroyed by it. Either someone is trustworthy or they're not, but being suspicious and controlling won't help. Remember: trust is the only basis for love.

Real love is hard work. There are times when your relationship feels impossible, right? When you look at other couples strolling hand in hand and think: *why can't we be like that?* But every relationship is a mystery from the outside. You never know what argument a couple has had before they turned up at the dinner party, what heartbreak may be bubbling beneath the surface or what ups and downs they've been through. Don't judge other couples' relationships, and don't compare your own. You have good times, too, when others look at you and think: *why can't we be as happy as they are?* And remember: real love is hard work. Just being in love isn't enough for a relationship to thrive; you also need to work on communicating, listening to each other, as well as being flexible, generous and patient.

The language of love. Everyone communicates differently. Women tend to be more emotionally and verbally expressive, whereas men often demonstrate their feelings through practical actions. Fixing your bike, or bringing home your favourite takeaway, can be as romantic as endless declarations of love: just expressed in a different way. Whether it's through words, actions or touch, accept that everyone says it differently.

Drama isn't the same as love. Fiery relationships are usually full of drama: passionate rows followed by passionate reconciliations. But don't confuse drama with love. Those rollercoaster emotions can get exhausting pretty quickly – for you and for everyone else around you. Constant rows are not a good basis for a long-term future. If you're constantly breaking up and then making up, you're probably incompatible.

When to give up. Sometimes two people aren't meant to be together. You can love someone with all your heart and still not be able to make it work: you're simply the wrong combination. Try a few times, by all means, but don't go on forever. Remember: love is not supposed to be painful. Walking away from a failing relationship is not a sign of weakness. It will save you so much heartbreak in the end. Letting go of someone can be the strongest thing you do.

Time out. Time apart is essential in any relationship; how much depends on you and your partner. Some people are naturally gregarious, whereas others prefer to interact in small groups or one-on-one. Some people are very sociable, but also need time alone to recharge their batteries. Make sure you get what *you* need, and respect your partner's needs too. Don't feel unwanted if they need time to themselves: needing solitude is not a personal rejection. Sharing a life doesn't have to mean sharing every single thing – it's healthy to have separate interests. Being apart can often make you stronger and more interesting when you come back together.

Relationships aren't the *solution*. If you're broken, being in a relationship won't fix you. If you're bored, lonely or unhappy, no one else can mend you. I always think of those lines in the movie *Jerry Maguire* when Tom Cruise tells Renée Zellweger: 'You complete me.' It's romantic – but you shouldn't be waiting around for another person to complete you. First of all, try being a whole person yourself. There is absolutely no point in being with someone because you're terrified of being alone.

Accept yourself. Single, married, cohabiting or whatever, no one has it all. The secret to staying sane, let alone content, must be to accept that nothing's perfect. Even the princess of pop, the beautiful, talented, millionaire singer Kylie Minogue, doesn't 'have it all'. In a 2015 interview with *Event magazine*, she said: 'I've got a really successful career but I haven't got everything. I haven't got the relationship. I haven't got children. It just didn't happen for me.'

Relationships with others are essential to human well-being, but romantic love can be challenging as well as rewarding. Finding someone else shouldn't become a fixation, and being single shouldn't be seen as an affliction. If you're enjoying dating, fine; if not, give yourself a break. You don't need that 'other half' to complete you: each one of us is a perfect, primal whole. Being alone can give you valuable time to develop and grow as a person. Learning to value and respect yourself, partner or no partner, is a crucial step on your primal journey.

Love

According to Aristophanes, humans were originally created as spherical hermaphrodites with four arms, four legs and two heads. Then, as a punishment for insolence, these beings were split in half by Zeus, and now we're wandering the earth with only two arms and two legs, effectively split down the middle and feeling incomplete. Aristophanes explains that 'human nature was originally one and we were a whole, and the desire and pursuit of the whole is called love' (Plato's *Symposium*).

This is why we talk about the search for love as 'looking for our other half', or trying to find the 'right person' for us. But it's not all about just one other person. From Plato to Eros, there are many kinds of love: platonic, erotic, filial, romantic and sexual. Think of the different feelings you experience for those who matter in your life: your boyfriend, girlfriend or spouse, your child, your parents, your best friend, even your pet.

And then there is love for the self: arguably the most important of all. Can one really love others until one has learned self-respect, self-esteem, and inner compassion and kindness? It's easy to care about others – but to treat oneself with the same respect and care is fundamental to a balanced, stable emotional state.

Why do we need love anyway – what are we looking for? We don't start life alone; we begin as part of another (our mother) and so we seek to recreate that feeling of belonging. In this way, love is deeply primal. The loss of that intimacy, that separation from the breast, is a traumatic rupture which we seek to heal by finding that closeness again in a life partner. There's no doubt that love is one of the most primal emotions we experience, but it can be hard to know why.

Primal Emotions

66 *Feeling lost, crazy and desperate belongs to a good life as much as optimism, certainty and reason.* 99
Alain de Botton

Pleasurable and painful, unpredictable and uncontrollable, confusing and life-changing: our deepest primal emotions are part of being human. Anyone who feels 'lost, crazy and desperate' should feel able to ask for help. But we must understand that life is full of ups and downs: difficult emotions are as much a part of human experience as joyful ones. Like light and darkness, yin and yang, everyone goes through good times and bad. Honouring those emotions, taking time to feel the pain as well as the happiness, is a fundamental part of this primal journey.

Negative experiences and emotions are often airbrushed out of modern society. With endless streams of perfect images showing off our fabulous lifestyles, it's easy to feel that you're the only one falling, failing or feeling depressed.

However, accepting that life is frequently imperfect is part of becoming a fully rounded human being. After all, if we've never struggled, how can we empathise with others? The recent focus on giving mental health parity of esteem with physical health is undeniably positive, but fixing broken hearts or heads is not as simple as fixing a broken leg. Not everything can be talked or medicated better.

If we want to cope with whatever life throws at us, we have to accept that we are not in control. We also have to stop feeling ashamed of negative emotions, hiding them, or blaming ourselves or others. Forget triathlons and travelling solo through Borneo: it can be far braver to face up to your own dark night of the soul and not give up.

The flipside of sadness is happiness – and it's important to celebrate this too. Research shows that we register pain more intensely than pleasure. When everything is going fine, we have a tendency to take it for granted. Contentment may not be dramatic, but it's also important. Just as mindful eating heightens the taste and texture of food, so being aware of positive emotions enhances them. These happy moments are rarely operatic sunsets or ecstatic epiphanies: in fact, they can be all the more intense for their simplicity. Next time you're sitting in a shaft of sunlight, or sipping a really wonderful coffee, take a moment to absorb the simple pleasure. Focus on the quality of that sensation: is it ease, warmth, anticipation? What does that moment of contentment feel like? Primal emotions, both negative and positive, deserve to be fully felt.

Other Primal Feelings

Love is only one of the instinctive emotions which we share with our distant ancestors. Emotions are one of our closest links with primal forebears. The external world may have changed out of all recognition since those caveman days, but deep inside us those primal feelings of fear, hostility, anger, hunger, sexual desire, aggression and protectiveness remain.

These emotions are as powerful as ever, but we're not very good at expressing them. From childhood we're taught to suppress our feelings: it's not manly to show fear, little boys are told; it's not ladylike to show aggression, little girls are told. It's not polite to react with anger when someone treats you unfairly or to lean over and caress someone because you find them sexually alluring. It's not appropriate to show hunger when you turn up at a party – you don't run over to the buffet and cram food into your mouth! So many emotions and urges, which we all experience and are socially conditioned to conceal.

Occasionally, the raw human emotions break through the carefully constructed politeness. This could be at times of intense pain or grief: a widow keening over the body of her dead husband, a woman in the throes of childbirth or a refugee family begging for asylum, for example. At such extreme moments, issues of cultural appropriateness become irrelevant. At the other end of the spectrum, the collective euphoria of a live football or boxing match can make crowds behave in ways that at any other time would be severely looked down upon.

Emotions are also cultural. The traditional Irish funeral wake, for example, includes rituals such as story-telling, singing and merrymaking. During the holy festival of Ashura, Shia Muslims beat their chests with chains and knives, some even gashing their heads, to reflect the suffering of the Prophet Muhammad's grandson. In Aboriginal cultures, mourners take part in symbolic chants, songs and dances, as well as painting and cutting their own bodies. When compared to the quiet British funeral service – usually hymns, readings from scripture and then burial or cremation – it's clear to see why we're considered reserved, even buttoned-up.

There are also generalisations about Southern European populations. From food to romance, Italians and Spaniards are considered to be far more passionate and demonstrative than their Northern counterparts. Some of these cultural stereotypes are outdated, while others hold true.

Emotions are a generational issue, too: during the twentieth century, the UK gradually became more emotionally open – *too* open, some might say. With the 'invention' of adolescence around the 1950s, and the development of psychology as a science of mind and behaviour, as well as rock and roll, drugs and free love, the emphasis shifted from keeping it in to letting it out. We have become a far more tolerant society, casting off many taboos around sexuality and race, for example.

From the reserve of the First and Second World War generations, who kept a lot of feelings inside, it's now de rigueur for most teenagers to have a blog or social media account, charting their everyday emotional highs and lows. My father, in his 80s, rarely talks about his *feelings*, and I've never seen him cry.

As with most human behaviour, there's a fine line to be drawn. Repressing intense emotions can be damaging, but letting it all hang out can also get you in trouble! Good manners and politeness – not screaming at the driver who cut you up on the motorway, for example – are important aspects of a civilised society. But keep too much bottled up inside and the situation will only get worse: have you ever remained silent during an unjust situation at work or in your personal life? Failing to speak up, or stand up for ourselves, makes us miserable too.

Emoji or Emotions?

In late 2015, Twitter issued this update: *hearts are the new high five. Or hug. Or thank you. Just tap the heart on any Tweet to instantly share how you feel, no matter what that is.*

Whether it's emojis, emoticons, thumbs up or 'like' or heart buttons, the Internet has a lot to answer for.

The smiley face icon, which began life in Japan in the 1990s, has become a global lingua franca. That original yellow emoji has spawned thousands of variants, expressing a vast emotional range stretching across happy, frustrated, nostalgic, confused, annoyed, hurt and tired. We're clearly desperate to express *something* from behind the safe barriers of our digital screens.

On social media, emojis say so much: celebrities post sad faces when break-ups are confirmed, steaming turds when they're having a bad day, baby emojis when they're announcing a pregnancy, or champagne when their song gets to number one. The British tennis player Andy Murray is known for being a man of few words. Fittingly then, on the morning of his wedding in April 2015 he tweeted a long string of emoticons (sunshine, showers, hairdressers, church, bride, ring, cameras, cake, cocktails, beer and dancing).

Sometimes, it seems, the more digitally fluent we are, the more inarticulate we become. Are our feelings of joy or sadness so difficult to communicate that we simply opt for a yellow face instead? Recent petitions for a 'dislike' button on Facebook, to indicate disapproval or non-agreement, could be seen as part of this general emotional inarticulacy. Whatever happened to saying it with words? Are our emotions not intense enough to matter or too intense to explain?

Understand Your Physiology

In order to express our feelings more articulately, it helps to understand what's going on inside. Your emotional state affects your physical state on every level: your psychological and physiological functioning are intimately linked. The body's physical response to emotions is deeply, inescapably primal, no matter how hard you try to hide or override it.

The body's key functions and emotions are regulated by the following systems.

Nervous system: with a network of around one trillion neurons, the nervous system connects the brain and spinal cord with the rest of the body, receives and processes information from the skin, muscles and joints, and regulates movement.

Endocrine system: glands that produce and secrete hormones which regulate the body's growth, metabolism, sexual development and function. At times of emotion or stress, the endocrine system responds by releasing different hormones, such as adrenaline, cortisol or endorphins.

Respiratory system: the main respiratory organs are the lungs, which regulate the process of inhaling oxygen and exhaling carbon dioxide. When emotionally affected, we may experience shortness of breath or hyperventilation.

Cardiovascular system: the blood circulatory system which delivers oxygen and nutrients to every cell in the body via the system of blood vessels, arteries and the main pump: the heart. Heartbeat and blood pressure often increase at times of intense emotion.

Reproductive system: controls the biological processes behind human reproduction. It is closely affected by emotional state: for example, prolonged stress can have an impact on women's menstrual cycles and men's sperm count, and therefore on the ability to conceive.

- **Immune system:** provides the body's resistance to infection and toxins. Ongoing stress places immune function under pressure, increasing the body's susceptibility to infection, slow wound-healing, skin conditions or allergies.

- **Digestive system:** controls the digestion of nutrients into the bloodstream, delivers them around the body and looks after the elimination of waste products. Emotional disruption can affect digestion, leading to symptoms of indigestion, nausea and gas. Emotions also stimulate the muscles of the intestines, resulting in diarrhoea or constipation. Prolonged stress can trigger irritable bowel syndrome or ulcers.

- **Musculoskeletal system:** the skeleton, muscles, joints and connective tissues which provide form, stability and movement to the body. In emotional states, your muscles tense up, ready to deal with any perceived danger. Extreme stress or anxiety can cause headaches, general muscular tension or neck, shoulder and back pain.

Tune In...

Experiencing your emotions in a more primal way means tuning into these powerful physiological systems. This isn't hard: when you listen to your body's signals, it will tell you exactly how you feel.

- **Anger.** Your body temperature will rise, your stomach will clench and maybe so will your fists (under the table!). You may want to shout or hit something/someone hard.

- **Fear.** You hold your breath or begin to hyperventilate, breaking out into a 'cold sweat'. Your heart rate increases. The tiny hairs which cover your body stand up on end: this is pure primal 'fight or flight' reaction.

Sexual desire. Physical desire manifests itself in increased heart rate and blood pressure, flushing of the skin, increased blood flow to the genitals, and increased arousal and sensitivity.

Nerves. This is different to fear, but has similar physical results. Have you ever been preparing to give a public speech, and your insides begin to churn and you feel like you might be sick? Extreme nerves activate the 'fight or flight' system, as with fear, when no concrete threat is present. That stress causes a rush of adrenaline that redistributes both water and blood flow. Your primal self is gearing up to fight or flee, but instead you have to speak to a roomful of people...

Fatigue. Strictly speaking, fatigue is not an emotion, but it's a powerful human sensation, and being exhausted definitely messes with your moods.

Primal Parenting

Parenting is a deeply primal issue: how to bring up children is fraught with practical, moral, financial and social questions and challenges.

According to the American Academy of Pediatrics, children spend an average of seven hours a day on various forms of entertainment media, including televisions, computers, smartphones and other electronic devices. In an ideal world, children would be brought up as primally as possible, the way that many of us remember from our twentieth-century tech-free childhoods: playing outside with neighbourhood friends, reading books or building fortresses under the kitchen table. Of course, that's pie in the sky and hopelessly anachronistic: many babies and toddlers are now more at ease with electronic devices than their parents are. Some young children are given smartphones when they start school, raising a whole other set of safety and social questions. Is it safe for children to be online, unsupervised? Then again, is it safe for them *not* to have a phone – and is it fair, if all their friends have phones and tablets, to deprive them? Also, let's not forget about educational issues, when so many lessons and homework assignments now depend upon Internet access.

Parenting is an intensely private matter, but it has also become a subject for moral judgement and social opprobrium. Tabloid newspapers feature 'irresponsible' parents who leave their children unattended in the car for a few minutes or feed them junk food. From diet to exercise, to education and the Internet, parenting isn't an easy job these days.

In recent years there has been a positive movement known as 'free-range' parenting, as a reaction to the 'helicopter' style of parenting. Where helicopter parents hover over children, scheduling endless after-school activities and playdates, free-range parents let children learn, experiment and work things out by trial and error. Free-range parents are controversial, because they allow their children to play outside or to walk to school alone – within safe parameters, of course. They don't fuss if children pick up food from the floor – and they don't ban gluten or sugar. Free-range parenting is a primal reaction to our fearful, safety-conscious society.

In the end, parenting is about balance. Yes it's a big bad world out there, but we have to accept that children cannot be wrapped in cotton wool forever. They shouldn't be exposed to dangerous situations, but they do need to learn about independence at the appropriate age. They shouldn't be playing computer games for hours on end, but neither should they be deprived of all the opportunities to learn and interact online. As long as they're eating well, getting their five fruit and vegetables a day, the occasional sweet treat won't harm them. For children, as for adults, moderation is the ideal solution.

Primal parenting comes down to trusting yourself and your child. It's about prioritising what really matters – raising a healthy, happy child – and not obsessing over the rest.

Primal Grief

Bereavement and death are defining experiences – perhaps *the* defining experiences of our lives.

No matter how rich or powerful we may be, death will come to us all in the end. And before it does, it will happen to those close to us. Yet we ignore it, fear it and pretend it won't happen – and when it does, we don't know what to do or say.

Thankfully, we don't encounter much death in our daily lives any more: children no longer routinely die in infancy, we're not sending our loved ones off to war, infectious disease, cancers and AIDS survival rates are up, and life expectancy is increasing every year. When a life ends, it's sanitised: the corpse is tidied away, often going from the hospital bed to the morgue to the undertaker and into a coffin without us seeing them one last time. We don't touch dead bodies; we don't wash or dress our loved ones as our grandparents and great-grandparents used to.

Where is the place for grieving in our society? Not only have we lost those rituals around preparing and laying out the body, but we have even lost the rites of mourning. Apart from at the funeral, no one wears black clothes; to do so would be seen as embarrassingly sombre. In our fast-paced, secular world, in which religion is increasingly irrelevant, death is an embarrassment. What do we say to others except maybe: 'I'm sorry for your loss'? Even on the over-sharing world of social media, death is largely absent. We see an endless stream of holiday, wedding and new baby photographs, but how often does someone post from a funeral or a wake? When a famous figure dies, and public 'tributes' are paid to the deceased on social media, it can seem inappropriate, even trite.

Most religions maintain strong mourning rituals, notably Islam and Judaism. The Jewish tradition has a clearly defined process: from Aninut, the period between death and burial, to the intense seven-day post-burial period of Shiva, through Shlosim for 30 days after burial, and the one-year mourning stage. There are precise instructions on everything from paying calls to bereaved relatives at home, bringing them meals of condolence, covering mirrors, lighting candles and saying prayers. With these gentle, ancient rituals, the family is guided through the initial shock of grief and eased back into the world. In our secular Westernised society, we lack this clear structure. The funeral service may be the closest we come to the person we have lost, and then we're left to get on with things. Most people are back at work the next day. Perhaps having more formalised rituals of death might help us to come to terms with the reality of loss. When Jews are sitting Shiva, the community is there to provide for their needs and to comfort them in their grief.

There are different kinds of death, of course, and different experiences of bereavement. Losing a young child isn't the same as losing an elderly relative, although both can be devastating, no matter what age they were. Loss is one of the most primal emotions any human being can feel; it reduces you to the state of a small child, lost in the wilderness, crying out for someone to look after you. Nothing prepares you for the finality of that loss, the inescapable fact of silence, that you can never see, talk to or touch your loved one again.

Like all primal emotions of loss and heartbreak, grief needs to be honoured. Honouring your loss, and feeling the depths of sadness, is part of the process of mourning and healing. Whether through private ritual or formal prayer, with or without religious faith, you can find your own way of remembering the person you loved. It could be a visit to their graveside, reading their favourite poem, listening to 'your song', talking about them with others or just keeping their photo close to you.

Remember that grief is natural, and it needs to be felt. It won't heal in weeks or months: the primal sadness will stay with you for a long time, perhaps forever. The hole that the loss creates can never be filled, but it will gradually change, and it will hurt less intensely. Time will turn raw grief and loss into a richer kind of love and thankfulness.

Perfectly Primal Relationships

As we've seen, relationships figure in many different ways in our lives: some virtual, some romantic, some companionable – sometimes easy, sometimes tricky. Whatever form they take, your relationships should be a pleasure. Not necessarily *all* of the time, but most of the time. Being with your closest friends or partner should make you happy. Feeling angry or tense should not be an everyday occurrence. You should feel valued and appreciated – even desirable once in a while!

The magazine *Marie Claire* asked a group of women over 100 years of age for their life and relationship advice. Many of them mentioned laughing lots, enjoying sex and celebrating the everyday. One elegant centenarian also said: 'I don't like stress. I can't stand arguing. If anybody is fussing, I'm gone. I like to be around positive people, people who lift you up not bring you down.' Every human needs good, caring relationships in their life. Friendship, camaraderie, kinship and love are important for our health and happiness. Confiding in others keeps us emotionally balanced, and physical intimacy keeps us connected. Good relationships are infinitely rewarding – and they don't have to be hard. The key is to work along primal principles of trust, honesty and respect.

However busy life gets, you can always put these principles into practice. You can make time for your family and friends when they need you. You can give back to your community and get involved with the place where you live. You can treat others as you would like to be treated, practise kindness and show forgiveness. You can take a positive, practical approach to problems, avoiding negativity and blame.

The most primal relationship of all is the one with yourself. How you feel inside really matters: it's responsible to look after your own mental and physical health, not selfish. The more you listen to and understand your own body, your emotions and needs, the better friend, partner or parent you can be for others. So nurture and respect yourself; remember that no one is perfect and forgive yourself just as you forgive others. Strong, honest relationships, within and without, are the foundations for your positive, primal future.

Chapter 4
Primal Fertility

Fertility should be the most primal process of all: the means by which human life is created and by which our species continues to evolve. Motherhood is seen as a natural destiny, the *raison d'être* of every woman, the innate biological expression of their femininity. Which makes it even sadder and more frustrating when fertility doesn't happen as it should.

The miracles of modern medicine and advances in assisted conception and *in vitro* fertilisation mean that infertile women have ever greater chances of getting pregnant. This is sometimes controversial, as with the 65-year-old German woman Annegret Raunigk, already a mother of 13 children, who went on to give birth to quadruplets in May 2015. The media debated endlessly over whether it was morally right, or physically safe, for women to be artificially impregnated in their 50s and 60s, long after the menopause.

Whatever the rights and wrongs of reproductive science, it's a complicated and hotly debated social issue. You can barely open a newspaper without seeing another alarmist headline about plummeting fertility rates, risks and warnings. It's startling how public this deeply private issue has become: what could be more personal to women than their wombs? If and when they get pregnant, where and how and why – surely these are questions for women, their partners and their doctors alone?

> M, in her early 40s, has been trying to conceive for nearly a decade. She says: 'I don't know what to think any more. I spent years being careful to prevent myself from getting pregnant, then I stopped and found that conception didn't happen after all. I feel like contraception gives us the illusion that we're in control of our fertility. Turns out, maybe we're not…'

It can be hard to accept that we're *not* in control. In a super-scientific world where we can cure, schedule or modify most things, and where there's a pill for every ill, getting and staying pregnant can be a random, mysterious process. For some couples it happens instantly, whereas for others never at all. Even with IVF, pregnancy is by no means guaranteed. It can be a heartbreaking and financially crippling failure, raising the hopes of women who try for years, without success, to conceive.

Keep Calm and Carry On...

Despite the health warnings and the scare stories, we all know women who have conceived in their 40s or got pregnant naturally after years of IVF, just as they'd given up. The best thing for fertility is being healthy and positive, and the worst thing is anxiety. A recent US study found a 29 per cent reduction in fertility in couples with high stress levels. So, if you're worried about fertility issues, ignore the panic and instead follow some sane, simple advice.

Tip-top Health

There are plenty of positive steps you can take to improve your chances of conception. Three of the most effective steps are:

- **Cut out smoking:** female smokers have been shown to have an older 'ovarian age' and significantly lower rates of success with IVF.

- **Ditch the alcohol:** studies found that women who do not drink alcohol conceive more quickly and have fewer miscarriages.

- **Cut down on caffeine:** caffeine is thought to interfere with conception. Drink no more than 200 mg a day; that's the equivalent of around three mugs of tea, two cups of instant coffee or one cup of filter coffee.

Sperm Matters

From a primal perspective, both egg and sperm need to be in the best possible shape before conception. Unfortunately, modern life, which for many of us runs on stress, caffeine, alcohol and radio waves, isn't always the most primal place to start. It's often assumed that infertility is a female problem, but it can be a male problem too. Around 30–50 per cent of infertility investigations uncover problems with sperm quality, so it's important that men also get checked out. Most fertility clinics conduct routine semen analysis at an early stage.

Overheating is known to damage sperm quality, so men should keep their testicles as cool as possible, avoiding saunas, tight underwear, cycling, and resting laptops on their lap and mobiles in their front pockets.

Men should also consider overhauling their diet, just as women do. Asparagus and broccoli contain zinc, which is essential for healthy sperm and prostate health, and eating a few Brazil nuts a day is highly recommended. Antioxidants and folic acid can also improve male fertility. Salmon is an excellent source of omega-3 fatty acids, an important building block for sperm. Processed red meat (e.g. salami), and excessive levels of saturated fats, butter and cheese have been linked to poorer quality sperm.

Medication/Infection

Some prescription medication can affect fertility, so talk to your GP if you're concerned about this. And don't forget that past infections or STDs in either partner can cause problems with conception, so you should have the basic sexual health screenings.

Believe in Yourself

As we've seen, anxiety can be counterproductive. Instead of feeling negative about not getting pregnant, try thinking positive. Focus on why you want a baby and how happy you'll be when (not if) it happens. Don't avoid friends who get pregnant, and don't despair. Most women get there in the end.

If you're open-minded, visualisation techniques are thought to be powerful. Visualise your womb as a warm, welcoming place for an embryo to implant. Think about your unborn baby; imagine yourself as a mother.

Keep Sex Fun

Trying to conceive can become an all-consuming obsession and depressing when it doesn't happen. Make sure you maintain other interests apart from having a baby, and share experiences, so that you and your partner don't feel like you're 'failing'. Also, never put your life on hold: book holidays, move house, change jobs and keep doing whatever you'd normally do.

While it's essential to understand when your body is fertile, don't over-schedule sex. This takes the fun and spontaneity out of it, and increases the pressure. Scheduling sex can also reduce your likelihood of conceiving, as the more sex you have, the more chances you have. Sperm can live up to 72 hours in a woman's body, so having sex two or three times a week should catch that fertile window.

Many fertility experts also advise women not to overshare intimate details about ovulation, temperatures and cervical mucus with their partners – this is important information for women, but can be off-putting for men!

> **"**
>
> **Dr Gillian Lockwood, Medical Director of the Midland Fertility clinic, advises:** 'Know your family history. Women inherit their fertility potential through the female line, so a strong family history of premature menopause (before 50), endometriosis, fibroids or polycystic ovary syndrome (PCOS) should alert you to seek investigations earlier if things aren't going to plan.'

Primal Body Basics

- **Weight:** women who are significantly overweight or underweight may experience irregular ovulation, difficulties conceiving or a higher chance of miscarriage. Male fertility is also affected by body weight, especially the production of healthy sperm.

- **Exercise:** it's important to be fit and active when trying to conceive, but it's not the time to take up strenuous exercise. Intense exercise can trigger the release of the stress hormone cortisol, which may impair fertility. From a primal perspective, your body needs to be nurtured and cared for in order to conceive. Gentle exercise will relieve stress and improve fertility: opt for low-impact activities, such as swimming, walking or yoga.

Finally, try to accept whatever comes your way. This is incredibly hard, but a baby is a blessing not a right. Your primal mindset will help here: you matter, whether or not you're a parent or a partner; you have value in yourself. From a primal point of view, remember that there are plenty (some might say, far too many) of little beings on the planet; not every human needs to reproduce.

If possible, try not to compare and despair. It may feel like every other woman can get pregnant and you can't – but this is not the case. Around 20 per cent of women aged 45 now do not have children, not all of them by choice. Becoming bitter, or hanging onto sadness, will only make things worse. Staying sane about fertility – and infertility – requires an open, philosophical mind, and a dose of primal practicality. Whether due to luck or fate, or simply because you're on this Earth for another reason, not getting pregnant does not make you any less of a woman. Not being a father does not make you any less of a man. There will be frustration and grief, but there will also be a time to move on.

Kim Cattrall recently spoke on Radio 4's *Woman's Hour* about being child-free and single at the age of 59. The *Sex and the City* actress said that being a mother is not just about giving birth: 'I am not a biological parent, but I am a parent. I have young actors and actresses that I mentor… There is a way to become a mother in this day and age which doesn't include your name on the child's birth certificate. You can express that maternal side, very clearly, very strongly. It feels very satisfying.'

There are many ways to find meaning in life, and childbearing is not the only path. Of course, the creative urge isn't the same as the biological procreative urge, but there are ways to express your caring, nurturing side. Life will present other opportunities, and while they may not be like motherhood, they will be significant too. What about starting a business or teaching? As an employer or educator you will be supporting others in valuable ways.

Remember that beautiful African proverb: 'It takes a village to raise a child.' There are informal alternatives to creating a child of your own: wonderful, generous alternatives. There are many ways you can look after young people, through volunteering, teaching or nursing. You might be an uncle or aunt to children, a godparent, or simply a really good friend.

There are also formal alternatives to becoming biological parents, such as fostering and adoption. Think of all the children on this planet who live in fear, hunger or poverty, or who have lost their own parents. The adoption process can be long and difficult, but caring for another's child is a beautifully positive act.

Whether or not you become a biological parent, adopt or foster, or teach or mentor, there are many ways to care for other human beings. If you don't have babies or children in your life, could you give some time to the elderly, frail or vulnerable? What about helping refugees in desperate circumstances, or caring for animals in need or the environment? After all, the world isn't only about us humans – there are other ways to contribute: whether by rehoming an abandoned puppy or conserving this precious Earth for future generations. Spending our time and energy fighting for endangered species or wildlife is arguably as important as adding to the global population!

Thinking about different forms of 'fertility' can help us to challenge the notion that a woman's intrinsic worth is bound up in her reproductive capacity (and by implication, her youth and attractiveness). The social expectations that a woman's biological destiny is to become a mother is outdated; this simply doesn't apply to all women. The same goes for men, who can be incredibly generous and caring without being fathers. In a primal sense, society should value non-parents as much as it values parents.

Ultimately, there are no rules about what we can do with the primal urge to nurture and protect. Creating a new life isn't the only way to be creative. Let's not obsess about biological procreation, and let's not ignore the many ways in which individuals can show love and care. Our daily habits and working lives can be incredibly fertile, from researching or campaigning, to writing or painting, to sowing and reaping, even to recycling and reusing. Of course, newborn babies are miraculous, but so are seedlings. Nurturing the planet in all its fragile diversity is a powerful way of expressing our primal humanity.

Chapter 5
Primal Work

66 There is no such thing as work-life balance.
Everything worth fighting for unbalances your life. 99
Alain de Botton

I love this statement. It turns on its head everything we've been taught to believe: that 'work' is the predator and your 'life' is the victim – or that achieving that elusive work-life balance is the key to perfect happiness. But ask yourself this: would you be content to spend the four or five decades of your working life in a job which starts at 9 a.m. and ends at 5 p.m., and which never troubles, disrupts or engages you beyond the strict parameters of your paid hours of employment? Or would you prefer to find something you care about so much that it naturally spills into the rest of your life?

Of course, it's not that simple. Most of us are not 'called' to pursue a burning passion: we feel our way from degrees or training to first jobs, and work out from there what interests us. If you want to become a priest, a ballerina or an astronaut, you have a clear vocation, possibly from an early age. For the rest of us, work pays the bills – sometimes it's fulfilling, sometimes it's a drag. For a moment, though, allow yourself to imagine: if you could do anything, what would it be?

What You Do Is Who You Are

Someone once told me: 'What you repeatedly do is what you ultimately become.' This applies to our professional lives: if you work in an accountant's office every day, eventually you're an accountant – no matter how passionately you dream of rescuing animals or singing at La Scala.

Procrastinating about the occasional tedious chore is one thing, but we shouldn't procrastinate over the things that matter. We do far too much 'putting off' of real life, deferring the fresh start until we're richer, or thinner, or we've achieved this, that or the other. Living primally forces us to confront these excuses, because it forces us to live in the here and now.

The circumstances will probably never be absolutely ideal, but the important thing is to begin. Just get started on whatever it is you need to do, whichever changes you need to make. Remember: how you spend your time is how you spend your life. Start living for today.

My friend Paul works in an investment bank. He's in his early 40s and already wealthy, with 'Vice President' embossed on his business cards. Every time we have a beer, he tells me how much he despises his job and how he should have pursued his dreams of being in a band.

'The work I do is boring and repetitive, essentially moving other people's money around and making more of it. But the remuneration is good, and it's enabled me to invest in various properties of my own. The thing is, now I have to service a lot of mortgages to keep the whole thing running – and to invest in more. I'm hoping to be able to retire by the time I'm 50...'

And then what? Start the band he dreamed of as a teenager, aged 50? Whenever you find yourself using phrases like: 'I have to do this job because...' or 'It will enable me to make enough money to retire early', warning bells should go off. Of course, there's a compromise between dreams and reality, between fulfilling our higher destiny and paying the bills. In this uncertain economic climate, we all need to be prudent about savings and pensions. Job security can feel precarious and career options limited. But don't kid yourself that you don't have a choice. As long as you're making decisions and setting priorities, you have a choice.

Paul's not the only one making excuses. According to the HR firm Investors in People, 60 per cent of workers are unhappy in their current jobs, while the Office for National Statistics reports that 17.4 million British workers are considering changing jobs this year. And yet somehow we're better at finding reasons why *not*, rather than reasons why *now*. Some excuses are valid, of course, but they're also negative and predictable – yes, we're all too stressed, busy or cash-strapped. But don't forget that you only have one life. Making excuses helps us to avoid risking our pride, our reputation, maybe failing, but they also prevent us from changing and growing.

Ultimately, it doesn't matter if you make excuses – sadly, no one's going to notice if you never produce that amazing work which is inside you. But you will know, and you may end up regretting it. Taking a primal approach means thinking hard about the way you spend your life, and deciding to do something authentic.

No one can tell you what work you want to do – that has to come from inside. If you feel aimless, or not drawn in any particular direction, then it's worth doing more research. Talk to helpful friends or family, consult experts, save up, retrain and do whatever you need to do.

Primal Pay

Recent figures reveal that the average salary of a FTSE 100 chief executive has now reached £5 million a year. According to a report by the High Pay Centre think tank, these individuals are receiving 183 times the average worker's annual salary of £27,000 in the UK. The situation is even worse in the US, where top earners bring home around 300 times the average worker's salary.

Have we gone mad? How can any single person, no matter how experienced or well-connected, be considered to be worth £5 million a year? How can any individual, no matter how many MBAs they may have, even feel able to accept 183 times that of another human being (who may well work twice as hard in far more stressful conditions)? How can they accept so many times more than what any reasonable person would need to live on?

Of course, you'll never catch them pocketing their millions in ready cash, because that's not how it works. Instead, these ludicrous pay packets are squirreled away into offshore funds, pension schemes, travel perks and Swiss chalets. The vast sums are rationalised using weasel words like *remuneration, shares, performance-related bonuses* and *compensation*. Compensation for what?

When my friend talks of his 'remuneration', I admit I feel angry. In terms of primal humanity, this kind of bloated, unnecessary 'remuneration' is revolting. In a world where millions of people still live with insufficient food, no homes and no shoes on their feet it's hard to see how anyone can justify these stratospheric levels of inequality.

Working to Live or Living to Work?

Does it matter if our working lives are boring, and we're only doing it for the money? Well, yes. In his 2007 book *Affluenza*, Oliver James describes this 'obsessive, envious, keeping-up-with-the-Joneses' epidemic which is making us depressed, anxious, addicted and sad. He explains how this obsession affects us:

'The great majority of people in English-speaking nations now define their lives through earnings, possessions, appearances and celebrity, and those things are making them miserable.'

When we are driven solely by wealth or status, we risk neglecting other fundamental human needs, such as creativity, collaboration, a sense of community, personal fulfilment and self-expression.

Job Satisfaction

The *Financial Times* journalist Lucy Kellaway podcasts regularly about office life and the meaning of work. In a story about a shoeshiner in the City of London, she relates the experience of having her shoes shined for the first time, and how she got talking to the shiner. Despite her discomfort in her 'liberal north London soul' at having someone else kneeling at her feet, it turns out the man absolutely loves his job.

He explained that he was autonomous, enjoyed chatting to his customers and derived pleasure from a job well done. A few days later Kellaway meets a female banker at a dinner party, who moans about the 'disillusionment and misery' of working in financial services: the regulation, the sexism, the office politics and the endless pressure. Kellaway concludes that she'd rather wield a can of boot polish than go into banking. In terms of work satisfaction, the shoeshiner had it nailed (excuse the pun).

If you haven't heard Lucy Kellaway's podcasts, they're well worth seeking out – you can listen to them on the *Financial Times* website or your podcast app.

Living Your Dream?

When it comes to following your heart and changing the world, you may recall the Stanford University speech given by Steve Jobs in 2005. The late co-founder of Apple famously told students at their graduation ceremony: 'Your work is going to fill a large part of your life, and the only way to be truly satisfied is to do what you believe is great work. And the only way to do great work is to love what you do. If you haven't found it yet, keep looking. Don't settle.'

That's all well and good – but we still need roads to be cleaned, bins to be emptied and incontinence pads to be changed. None of this is classified as 'great work', but it's important, essential – even satisfying. Plenty of very worthwhile work is repetitive and relatively simple. Up to a third of all jobs in the British economy are classed as 'low-skilled' – and yet these jobs matter too. These millions of people are not necessarily driven by a creative calling, or pursuing an inner vocation, but simply carrying out work that needs doing. We'd quickly notice if these millions of workers decided not to turn up. Whether it's classed as high-skilled or low-skilled, work can be worthwhile and enriching in a primal sense.

Steve Jobs is inspiring, but he's speaking to the privileged few. Clearly, we need balance in our attitudes to work: a bit of Jobs-style idealism and a bit of reality. Any job, no matter how 'low-skilled' or mundane, can be done with pride. I've worked as a waitress and as a nanny, I've changed beds and pulled pints – I enjoyed all these jobs in their own ways, mostly for the people I got to meet. I remember my big brother working on rubbish trucks for Camden Council during his university holidays: he came back with fascinating stories of the other guys in his 'gang' and their skilful strategies for clearing each street quickly. Read George Orwell's *Down and Out in Paris and London* to see just how interesting some of these jobs can be!

These jobs weren't about self-expression; they simply enabled us to pay the bills, make money to travel or cover student debts. Whatever you're doing, even if it's not your 'dream', can be done with dignity and a smile. After all, there's a great difference between an excellent nurse, carer or binman and a sloppy one. This is work in the most primal sense: and in that sense can be deeply satisfying. The scandal is that we pay these essential workers so poorly.

Money or Meaning?

Are we looking for money or meaning – or both? The philosopher Roman Krznaric examines how our attitudes to work have changed over recent decades. In his book *How to Find Fulfilling Work* (2012) he points out that for centuries most people worked simply to provide food and shelter, so they didn't have time to worry about self-expression. However, with increasing prosperity, we now demand so much more from our employment: 'We've entered a new age of fulfilment, in which the great dream is to trade up from money to meaning.'

He's right. It used to be enough to get filthy rich: now we want to make a meaningful impact on the world, too.

Clearly, we need to rein in our expectations. We need to find a compromise between short-term pain and long-term gain. Can we live more intensely in the present, with meaningful work, while still keeping a roof over our heads? Tricky, but not impossible.

> ❝ *Without ambition one starts nothing.*
> *Without work one finishes nothing.*
> *The prize will not be sent to you. You have to win it.* ❞
> **Ralph Waldo Emerson**

It's important to have aspirations *and* to make plans – nothing comes to us on a plate, and setting targets can be hugely motivating. If you're a student, it's crucial to focus on your long-term goals: studying the right subjects, getting onto the right courses, pursuing the best work experience opportunities. Training to be a doctor or a lawyer, for example, takes many years of dedication and hard work: short-term sacrifice for long-term success.

But not to the exclusion of living our lives now. Today is really all we have. Remember: living (and working) primally means focusing on the here and now. Try thinking differently about the way you spend your working days.

- Do you feel your work has meaning?

- Are you helping others?

- Does it make a difference to the world around you, your community – are you contributing?

- If you were told you had only a year to live, would you continue doing this work?

- What might you do instead?

Make That Change

It's natural to get irritated with colleagues or frustrated with one's work from time to time – we all do. No one loves every minute of their jobs – there are always tedious parts of earning a living: that's why it's called labour. But if you find yourself regularly coming home and complaining about your job, or if it's making you very stressed or depressed, it could be time to reconsider. Ask yourself the following questions.

- Are you annoyed with having to work in general or is it your work specifically bringing you down?

- Can you see things changing anytime soon?

- Is there something else you feel drawn to do?

Spend a few months at least investigating alternative options, talking to others who have made similar moves and thinking seriously about the consequences of leaving your current employment. If you really want to change your working life, be honest with yourself.

- What are your essential financial commitments? These will include rent or mortgage, food, utility bills and childcare payments.

- What could you cut back on? These might include non-essentials like holidays/travel, cars, eating out, shopping, gym, Cable/Sky subscriptions, etc.

🌿 If you cut back on non-essential or discretionary costs, how much could you save?

🌿 Would this enable you to change jobs, retrain or go freelance?

When I first started writing, I was able to switch my mortgage payments to interest-only, for a limited period, to ease the transition from salaried 9–5 work into self-employment. This should only ever be a short-term option – and is entirely dependent on your mortgage provider and your individual circumstances – but it did take the financial pressure off while I was establishing a different source of income.

And remember that learning to compromise is essential: revolutions rarely happen all at once. If you can't change your work immediately, what about part-time options or volunteering? You could devote your Sunday afternoons, say, to the work you're passionate about. Shadow someone to gain an insight into the day-to-day roles and make useful contacts. Training courses are increasingly delivered online these days: could you study for qualifications in your evenings and weekends?

If you answer every one of these suggestions with 'I can't because...' then it's time to be honest with yourself. Do you really want to change?

As well as compromising, you might have to swallow your pride. It can be hard, if you're already senior in your field, to start afresh. Remember leaving primary school as one of the 'big' girls or boys and then starting in a secondary school right at the bottom? It can also be hard to convince people, if you're older, highly paid or qualified, that you want to get work experience.

But it's not impossible. These days everyone is working longer, and the workforce is becoming increasingly more varied and diverse. Talk to everyone you know, put the word out that you're looking for experience or part-time work. Above all, show willing and work hard. Primal work is all about throwing yourself in, body and soul. Forget about pride, pay grades or being too old to start over.

It's quite common for students to take a gap year before they embark on university and the rest of their lives. However, increased life expectancy (and job insecurity) means that our careers are longer and less certain than ever before. There's a growing trend for mid-life gap years, sabbaticals, retraining and changes of career at all ages.

It makes a lot of sense to stop and take stock every decade or so. Few of us are the same people we were at 18 or 21; our interests and skills evolve, as do the industries we work in. Someone who went into the 'Information Technology' sector 20 years ago will now be working in a completely different industry. The same goes for developments in publishing, marketing, music, teaching and science.

As people and workers, we change too: children, marriage, divorce, illness and financial circumstances will affect our options and priorities. We might not even know what we're good at after years in one industry. Maybe we should all take time out to travel, retrain or try new things. Perhaps everyone 'arty' could learn something practical – I've always liked the idea of carpentry – or those in the science fields could try writing a short story or putting on a play. Who knows what hidden talents we might discover?

If you're determined to plough your own furrow, success is far from guaranteed. You'll probably need to do other more practical work in order to finance your creative efforts. As well as finding a way to pay the bills, you'll also need to make an important decision early on: not to fear failure.

Think positive: a 'no' is just a delayed 'yes'

Did you know that Iris Murdoch's first *five* novels were rejected or that William Golding's *Lord of the Flies* was discarded as 'an absurd and uninteresting fantasy which was rubbish and dull'?

Luminaries from James Joyce to Judy Blume were repeatedly turned down; Marlon James, winner of the 2015 Booker Prize, received 78 rejections for his first novel.

Any struggling writer seeks comfort in the famous failures: it's the most primal source of inspiration. If they can fail again and again and not give up, if they can persevere against all odds and eventually succeed, so can you. It happens in every sector, from business to theatre, art and politics. To return to Steve Jobs, his early, ignominious sacking from Apple, before his eventual world-conquering reincarnation as the Apple saviour, has provided inspiration to digital entrepreneurs throughout the industry.

Whatever your field, seek out inspiring examples of failures who became successes. The Americans tend to be much better at embracing failure than us Brits. Whereas they view it as a lesson, and a stepping stone to success, we see it as, well, failure. They have delightful mantras, such as: 'When you fail, fail forward.' Your primal mindset will help you here: how would man have invented tools or fire if they hadn't tried out lots of other things first?

All of this means that we can't just wait around for success to strike. Working primally means getting stuck in, putting in the hard slog, whatever it takes to get your project off the ground. A chef I know who runs a successful online catering business started out having to cook every dish in his own kitchen, then get on his moped and deliver them himself. He now has ten staff working for him, but at the very start it was just him and his girlfriend. Things don't just 'happen' – we make them happen.

A turning point for me came when I got sick of making excuses. I realised that while I was moaning about being 'too busy' to write, what with my 'full-time job' and all, other people were out there making it happen. Others with full-time jobs were getting up at 5 a.m. and writing. In my last book, *Letting Go*, I explained how I stopped making excuses, faced my fears and finally got started on making my dream come true.

I always told myself that one day I'd be a writer but the years went by and still I wasn't writing. I repeated all the usual justifications to myself – lack of time, lack of resources, lack of ideas – but I began to see that these were just excuses. Whenever I did start writing, a few chapters of a novel here, a draft of an article there, I quickly became discouraged and gave up. Like any other occupation, writing requires practice, practice and more practice. Because I loved reading, I assumed I should be 'good' at writing, even though I really hadn't put the effort in.

Finally, something clicked. I began getting up a few hours before starting work and sitting at my desk, trying to get words down on the page. Sometimes the pages stayed blank; often they were covered with a lot of bad stuff... I tried not to read back over what I had written and just kept going instead, and eventually I improved. I got a few articles into the papers, which led to a weekly column in *The Times*, and I had my first book accepted for publication soon after that.

For me, starting to write stirred something very primal inside. There was – and still is – plenty of self-doubt but finally I was pursuing my dream, rather than just dreaming it. Writing, like many jobs, involves constant failure and rejection, but it's worth it. Listen to your heart and brain: what do you really want to do? Make a list, a sketch, a plan; take a few steps in the right direction and then start doing it.

And do it *before* you do anything else. There's something deeply primal about prioritising your own work first thing. Getting up early was exhausting, but satisfying. I may have yawned for the rest of the day, but it was better than feeling stuck and frustrated.

Work may be tiring, but it shouldn't be painful! Ideally, you'll feel interested and involved in the field in which you work. If not, take a look at what's going on. It might be a specific problem – say an unpleasant colleague, a difficult project or a long commute – in which case you can start looking for similar jobs in a different company or location. But if you really hate your work – or, as my friend said, 'feel I'm wasting my life', you need to think hard about a new direction. Time to get primal and think about what you're really on this Earth for. Face up to your own excuses. Stop fooling yourself.

Working Differently

> ❝ *I do work that takes a lot of focus at a standing desk that has a small treadmill under it, on a computer that doesn't have an email application. Walking slowly while I work has a lot of positive outcomes: one of them is that it more or less chains me to my desk. I put my phone in do-not-disturb mode and close any unnecessary applications or windows that are open on my computer. I put on my noise-cancelling headphones and play my "listen while writing" playlist.* ❞
> **Christine Carter, www.positivenews.org**

Now that's a woman who has confidence in her own working style! Primal working is about finding out how you function best and, wherever possible, incorporating that into your daily routine.

Standing desks are seeing a resurgence in popularity, although the practice has been around for decades. I was drawn to the idea when I discovered that my great-aunt, Virginia Woolf, used to write *standing up*, just like her older sister, the artist Vanessa Bell, who stood painting at her easel. Researchers have found that children learn better while standing, paying attention more closely and engaging more actively.

Standing desks, especially those with treadmills underneath, can seem a health craze too far. But who's to say that sitting for eight or nine hours at a desk is any less crazy? The human skeleton is designed to move around on two legs, rather than sitting hunched up on its tailbone. If I've been sitting at my desk writing for too long, I become progressively more hunched over, shoulders tensed up, spine curled. A friend (also a writer) tells me she ends up in the shape of a prawn!

Even in the most ergonomic office chair, sitting for prolonged periods of time can be damaging for the following reasons.

🌿 It tightens up the hips and lower back.

🌿 It atrophies the walking muscles.

It increases compressive forces through the spine by 50 per cent, compared to standing.

It distorts the spinal curve and creates muscular imbalances.

It increases the risk of back pain, diabetes and heart disease.

If standing desks haven't reached your workplace yet, make sure you stand up and walk about regularly during the day, at least once every half an hour. This will reset your spine, and improve your oxygen, lymph and blood flow. Above all, avoid working in exactly the same position hour after hour and day after day: check your posture, vary your position and keep moving. By avoiding sameness, you'll keep bad habits at bay.

A Room of One's Own

Formerly known as the man-cave, now it's all about the 'she-shed'.

From small businesses to home gyms, photographic studios or yoga retreats, places to bake or sew in, or to throw children's parties or even as a spare bedroom, the shed has become the new female creative domain.

It used to be a safe haven in the garden where henpecked husbands could retreat to tinker with their tools, but it appears that women are reclaiming this outdoor sanctuary. In August 2015, the papers reported that shed purchases in the UK had risen by 50 per cent, with sales driven mostly by women.

Unlike male sheds, women's tend not to be filled with broken lawnmowers or build-your-own shortwave radios. Female sheds cover a range of outdoor constructions, from chic shaker-style summer houses to fully functional offices, to cosy, private dens. Shed offices can also be practical for those who need to juggle family life with running their own business.

One of my friends, a former ballerina, runs her Pilates studio from her garden shed – although 'shed' seems rather a humble label for her elegant wooden cabin containing ballet barre, full-length mirrors and sauna. As well as using it for her teaching, we often escape there with a bottle of Sauvignon Blanc.

Another friend, this one an interior designer, has built a stunning glass studio in her Japanese-style garden. I have borrowed it to write in sometimes... Looking out on the white gravel, bonsai trees and carp-filled pond, I feel more than a pang of shed-envy.

Gender aside, sheds are a great solution to working from home. Whether it has high-speed broadband, high-spec recording equipment and a fridgeful of beer, or a comfy old sofa and a pile of magazines, there's something wonderfully primal about being in a small construction in the outdoors. No commute, train strikes or traffic jams: walking out of your house and down the garden to work (ideally barefoot) feels positively primal.

Working hard for something you don't care about is called stress; working hard for something you love is called passion.

It's estimated that around 4.2 million people work from home in the UK. From personal experience, one of the hardest things about going freelance was losing that daily office camaraderie; working alone can make you feel directionless and out of the loop. However, being self-employed doesn't have to mean working alone: these days, many freelancers are choosing to gather with others. With the rise of remote working, freelancing and the 24–7 smartphone culture, the old office model is looking increasingly outdated. Many entrepreneurs, especially when they're starting out, hire desks in shared workspaces: with office facilities and meeting rooms, these shared work hubs are a useful way to run a small business without the risk and overheads involved in committing to larger premises.

Did you know? More than half of the new jobs created in the UK since the economic downturn of 2008 have been on a self-employment basis. The Royal Society for the Encouragement of Arts, Manufacture and Commerce predicts that the number of self-employed workers will overtake those employed in the public sector by 2018.

Along with this move away from fixed office spaces, is the awareness, central to living more primally, that we don't necessarily want to spend five of our seven days a week confined to a building, chained to a desk, staring at a screen, clocking in and clocking out. Digital technology is a mixed blessing in the world of work: while it enables us to work anywhere, at any time, it also means that we rarely disconnect completely. At the heart of primal working is finding a way to make this technology work for you: giving you the freedom to work more flexibly, without it becoming a ball and chain.

You might think that regularly disconnecting, as advocated throughout this book, would be detrimental to your career prospects, maybe even your social life. You'll be offline and out of the loop, right? On the contrary, disconnecting is very good for your work. It promotes original thinking and enables you to get a fresh perspective. Exploit the opportunities online, by all means, but don't let it overwhelm you. Don't forget, occasionally, to switch off the smartphone and go for a walk. Stay human: stay primal.

Technology overload is not the only challenge when you're working alone. If you're self-employed or working from home, you may find it hard to keep yourself motivated. Good time management sounds dull, but it's essential to maintaining a positive work-life balance, in or out of the office. Although adapting to life without external targets, deadlines or end-of-year appraisals can be tough, here are some tips for staying focused and managing your workload.

- Make a list of everything you need to do at the start of each working day. Number the list according to priority levels: 1 being the most urgent task and 10 being the task that can wait.

- Always start with the most urgent task, and don't do anything else until this is complete. However you accomplish this – whether it's turning off emails and phone alerts, shutting yourself in the 'quiet office' or not allowing yourself a coffee until it's done (my preferred tactic) – just don't let other distractions prevent you from tackling the number 1 task.

Don't expect to have everything finished by the end of each day. Transfer the not-yet-completed tasks to a fresh list the following day.

Making a list can help you to deal with that sense of overload: seeing all the jobs clearly set out will free up your mind and help you focus on your priorities: what needs to be done now and what can wait.

Even if you don't have a formal appraisal – or the financial incentive of a performance-related bonus – there are other ways to keep yourself on track. You could pair up with a fellow self-employed friend to set aims and objectives. Talk to others in the same sector and attend industry events or conferences. Find a mentor or organise meet-ups: the key here is to stay connected to others. This will avoid isolation and keep you enthusiastic about your work.

The Sharing Economy

From people sharing cars, delivering parcels for others, recycling unwanted furniture or renting out their homes, the sharing economy is spawning new ways to live, earn and consume in the twenty-first century. After decades of big business and global brands calling the shots, this is an exciting grassroots movement, fuelled by the rise of the Internet and smartphones. It consists of ordinary people making money from their skills and interests, from things they already own, or items that they want to rent out, share or give away.

The sharing economy is overturning the traditional model of consumerism, transforming the way we buy and sell, and replacing financial transactions with more personalised experiences. Also called a revolution of kindness, the sharing economy is changing the way we live, work and consume. It's green, it's sociable and it's flexible. It's also profitable: the accountancy firm PricewaterhouseCoopers has forecast that the 'sharing economy' will grow from around £500 million to £9 billion over the next decade.

Nimber launched in the UK in July 2015, describing themselves as 'social delivery service where you save the environment, make money and do something nice for other people'. It *is* nice to transport someone else's precious goods, save unnecessary transportation costs and pollution, and earn some cash into the bargain. It's similar to carpooling, which sadly never spread as widely as it might have, as we still see so many cars carrying just one or two people. Uber is also picking up on the idea of 'social delivery', with cargo vans and bikes sharing space with goods to be delivered, and a new taxi-pooling scheme to cut the cost of journeys – and congestion and pollution too.

Streetlife.com

The Internet also brings people together closer to home. Until recently I wasn't involved in my local community and knew hardly any of my neighbours (which is typical of many Londoners, but it's also a shame). Then I joined Streetlife.com, which claims to have over a million users across the UK, with community boards and discussion forums, and it's great fun!

It's simple enough – you enter your postcode and they connect you with others 'talking, sharing and caring' in your neighbourhood. The conversations in my area range from the sublime to the informative to the ridiculous: everything from wanting to start a cake business to lost cats and car keys, saving libraries and pubs, organising community clean-ups, taking action on persistent car alarms or finding a good Catholic church. There's someone giving away six baby spider plants, another wanting to borrow a ladies' bike for a month and even a skilled carpenter who requires meditation lessons in return for doing odd jobs.

Sharing cars or pressure washers means more use and less waste. Why shell out for a lawnmower when you could borrow one from a neighbour a few doors away? I've given away weatherproof and gloss paint (after using only half the amount I'd bought) and ended up becoming friends with the woman I gave it to.

Streetbank is another successful tech initiative. It has around 64,000 members worldwide, allowing neighbours to share stepladders, hedge cutters and similar resources but, more importantly, to connect. There's no commercial gain (except for the savings everyone makes) but there's a real benefit to individuals, communities and the environment. Everything about these green, friendly ventures makes sense: why shouldn't we share as much as we shop?

Green, sustainable, eco-friendly forms of living are often dismissed as unprofitable, even anti-capitalist. However, there is no reason why being green has to mean being poor. Whether it's reusing and recycling on a local scale, or developing truly sustainable energy on a national and international scale, this could be the shot in the arm which the global economy needs. As the world's ever-expanding population constantly requires more power, more water, more food, the demand is guaranteed. And if we can find a way to make renewable natural resources reliable, the potential for profit is limitless.

We're not there yet – but it's not impossible. It starts with green initiatives in our homes, our neighbourhoods and our regions; it begins with every one of us acting local and thinking global. Finding green sources of energy will take commitment, investment and determination in the short-term, but it will pay off in the long term. If we can put humans on the Moon, we can find a way to harness wind, wave and solar energy for the good of everyone on Earth. And there's no doubt that sharing our goods and skills, cutting down on waste, reusing, and recycling are all positive, primal ways to start.

The Gig Economy

Linked to sharing and caring is another sector known as the 'gig economy'. This is made up of those convenience-based, time-saving services which are fast becoming a part of our daily lives: ever had a hairdresser, masseur or manicurist come to your home? How about finding a local plumber or cleaner online, ordering an Uber, or using a delivery courier to pick up a package? The gig economy is all about connecting individuals who need something done with others who can do it.

It's less overtly altruistic than the sharing economy – the skills and services are not free – but there are overlaps. Compared to the traditional model of big business, this is on a more human scale, often dependent on local recommendations or online customer ratings. It won't come as a surprise then that in the economic uncertainty and job insecurity of recent years, this ad hoc sector is on the up and up. Professionals, from nail technicians to tax advisers, only need an Internet connection in order to set up their own business. This sector thrives on the proliferation of freelance work, the speed of online technology and the shared office hubs springing up around the country. It's bespoke, it's flexible and it benefits your community.

Whether it's local decorators or gardeners, a part-time hairdresser or Pilates teacher, this model of informal employment is friendly and green. It's also far more primal, returning us to times when people shared what they had, and when each individual's skills and services were truly valued. After all, money is only useful for what it can buy: if you're able to exchange a haircut from a local hairdresser for your skills as a decorator, cold hard cash becomes less essential. Of course, we're nowhere near the end of money, but the rise of the sharing and gig economies is a welcome reminder that humans are worth more than simply what it says on our bank balances. In a primal sense, we all have something to contribute.

Opportunities Online

With the rise of the Internet and growing numbers of freelancers, the opportunities for going it alone are greater than ever. The web-based marketplace is booming, with individuals able to sell their goods and services online. Etsy is an example of a website which opens up a whole world of possibilities for small creative ventures.

> **Becky, 29, fashion designer:** I buy old clothes from vintage shops and second-hand stalls, and make them into evening dresses. I started off doing it in my spare time but things have been taking off. For now, I have to keep my day job (in marketing) but the dream is to make dresses full-time… I'd never be able to afford rent on a shop, but on Etsy I have customers all over the world. A woman in California bought one of my dresses and then recommended me to her friends. The Internet has made all this possible.

Although the digital revolution has been democratising, it has also made life difficult for the self-employed, as it can be increasingly hard to 'monetise' your work. Writers and journalists are constantly being asked to write 'a few lines' for free, while designers and artists are asked to provide unpaid samples – and if we question this model of working for nothing, we're told that it's 'good publicity'. A friend who is a professional photographer says he really struggles 'because everybody has a camera-phone these days'. His years of experience in the industry, his media contacts and technical skill, of course, keep him in work, but there's no doubt that the ubiquity of images of any public event makes his job that much harder. Musicians are feeling the strain too, with so much music now available online for free. Taylor Swift, the multi-millionaire singer, recently stood up to Apple, as they launched their new music streaming service, demanding that they 'pay me if you want to play me' – and she triumphed.

Chances are that whatever you want to do will be competitive – after all, interesting people want to do interesting things! You need to make a pact with yourself, from the outset, not to give up. It will involve self-belief, inspiration, commitment and all that... but mostly it will involve hard work.

Reality Check

Where do you stand on money matters? If you're primarily motivated by salary, that's fine – but be clear with yourself about this. If your priorities include a large house, new car and regular foreign holidays, there is little point in writing novels.

Society romanticises creativity – the scribbling poet, the entre-preneur's eureka moment, the starving artist in the garret – but the reality is that these creative types are mostly very poorly paid. A survey in 2013 found that the median income of professional authors was £11,000 – nearly £6,000 below what the Joseph Rowntree Foundation considers necessary for a minimum standard of living. The average musician or artist earns even less. Those well-known success stories who make millions from chance discoveries – J. K. Rowling's *Harry Potter* series after years of poverty as a single mother, for example – are vanishingly rare: the majority barely scrape minimum wage from their self-expression. You may have to be prepared to temp or take part-time jobs to pay the bills.

There are plenty of business manuals out there which promise to help you make your first million while sipping cocktails on a Caribbean island, working no more than four hours a week and joining the ranks of the super-rich. However, most of us know that work is work, no matter how creatively fulfilling, and it takes effort. 'Overnight success' usually takes many years to achieve. It's unlikely you'll get anywhere on your own by only working four hours (or even four days) a week. Generally, you get out what you put in.

A Word About Money

Research shows that money matters. There is no doubt that interning is a great way to gain experience, and volunteering is a noble and satisfying endeavour, but nonetheless, paid work matters. Not just to pay the bills, but also for our psychological health and self-esteem. Studies in occupational psychology have found that being paid for what we do actually triggers the release of dopamine in our brains and gives us a sense of purpose. This explains why women who give up paid employment to become stay-at-home mothers often feel undervalued, even invisible. Being at home with children and running a household is most certainly hard work, but it is not financially recognised as such. Daniel Freeman, Oxford professor of clinical psychology and co-author of *The Stressed Sex*, explains why unpaid work makes us feel worthless. 'Whatever you do, you want to be recognised. Any situation where that doesn't happen puts you under stress, you feel less valued, and it chips away at your self-esteem.'

That said, financial payment isn't the only way to feel appreciated: many volunteers derive great satisfaction from the work they do without money changing hands. Contributing to society, helping the vulnerable, and giving one's time, expertise and care can be genuinely rewarding. Primal work can be paid or unpaid, but it should give us a sense of purpose. Being made redundant, even retiring, can trigger depression; many unemployed people struggle with the lack of purpose that not having a job can bring: a sense of feeling left out, irrelevant.

It's a natural human impulse to want to feel useful: to contribute to the world and to have our efforts valued. Nevertheless, many workers in our society go unrecognised. It's essential that we should value and reward those who do the hardest work of caring and nursing, often with little recognition or support, and frequently on the minimum wage. In a primal sense, these workers are the most important in our society, not the least.

Primal and Successful?

You may think that taking a primal attitude to work precludes being wealthy and ambitious – but that's not the case. You can be a hugely successful entrepreneur while still maintaining your human values, respecting the planet and keeping it primal.

The founder of Tiger stores is an excellent example. Lennart Lajboschitz is not a household name, but his empire spans 467 shops across 26 countries (with 46 of those in the UK). Described as the high street's answer to Ikea, Tiger sells everything from selfie sticks to mugs to umbrellas – functional, everyday items at very low prices. It has made the Danish entrepreneur a millionaire many times over.

Do we need any more of this cheap, disposable junk? Being primal is about buying less, reusing more and valuing what we already have. But Lajboschitz is an interesting example of a businessman who really cares about social interaction and human happiness. He sees himself as an anthropologist rather than a retailer, making functional products into emotional products, and aiming to bring people together and spread pleasure around the world. It's an interesting business example of how successful can be human; commercial can be primal, too.

Work-life Balance

For all that I've said about making your work your life, there is still a balance to be struck between employment and enjoyment. Working hard is one thing, but overdoing it simply risks stress and burnout. In the 1930s, the economist Maynard Keynes predicted that we would be working just three hours a day by now. In fact, the opposite is true: in Britain the average working week is 42 hours. But it seems that quantity does not always equal quality: despite UK working hours steadily increasing, we're one of the least productive countries in Europe.

Clearly, there is a balance to be struck between personal and professional, and it's this balance which is at the heart of primal work: putting the hours in and getting the job done to the best of your abilities, but knowing when to stop. It's hard, particularly if you're self-employed or work from home, to maintain that equilibrium between work and real life, family, friends and time for yourself.

However, finding this balance is essential to your primal well-being. Endless studies have shown that employees who exercise and make time for a personal life are happier, healthier and more efficient. In every sector, from computer programming to long-distance lorry driving to air traffic control, research shows that long hours lead to tired, accident-prone brains. We know this from our own experiences too: time away from the computer is valuable time to recharge, so you can return to your work with renewed vigour. You may be able to pull 17-hour days for a while, but not forever.

All Work and No Play...

While we should always take pride in our jobs, whatever we do, all work and no play can make life dull indeed. Work has its place, but so does time spent not working, networking or emailing, maybe not even concentrating. The modern obsession with productivity and profit can go too far, and sometimes we forget the joy of doing nothing much at all.

Idling, as extolled by the eighteenth-century writer Dr Samuel Johnson, and more recently by Tom Hodgkinson (editor of *The Idler* and founder of the Idler Academy) also has great merit. It is intensely primal, in all its forms: from reading to chatting to wandering to just gazing into the distance. Idling is the perfect counter-balance to the careerist, ambitious always-connected world of work. It gives us an excellent perspective too: after all, what was work originally for?

Idling is also good for you. There is overwhelming evidence that a lifetime of stress and overwork is damaging to both physical and mental health. The competitive corporate world, with its increasingly longer hours and shorter holidays, barely noticeable maternity leave and non-existent lunch breaks, isn't always a happy place to be. The growing tendency towards reification within the workplace – treating employees like units on a spreadsheet, measuring their value in terms of output and productivity – is intensely un-primal. Corporate jargon such as 'human resources' is dehumanising in a similar way: what is wrong with using terms like 'personnel', 'staff' or even 'workers'? Politicians are endlessly harping on about 'hard-working families'; we're bombarded with financial headlines about profitability, increased GDP and annual growth; we accept that salaries must increase, companies must expand and economies must grow – but why?

Perhaps you know those lovely lines from W. H. Davies's poem 'Leisure': 'What is this life if, full of care, We have no time to stand and stare.' Once in a while we need to step back and ask ourselves a few primal questions: what do I have? What do I need? What is work for? If we're able to provide food, clothes and shelter – if we're able to live well and enjoy the occasional treat – isn't that enough? Our brief spell on this Earth cannot just be about accumulating wealth and acquiring goods. We also need time for living and loving and daydreaming.

Idling is a joyous, primal habit. Whether it's zoning out for a few minutes in the office, gazing out of the window or taking an aimless stroll at lunchtime, both your brain and body benefit from those idle moments. Humans are not designed to concentrate for prolonged periods and we cannot constantly be firing on all cylinders. We need variety, interruption and surprise to keep us fresh. Primal work, paradoxically, requires primal play. Our minds naturally switch between focusing and floating. Modern workplaces militate against idle time, but it can be more productive than we realise.

Your primal journey is all about balance, so don't forget the balance between productive work and delightful, playful idleness.

Rethink

There's a beautiful line from the poet Mary Oliver that I have on my study wall:

> 66 *Tell me, what is it you plan to do*
> *With your one wild and precious life?* 99

What if you could start thinking differently about your work and how you spend your days? What if the metric of success could be enjoyment and freedom instead of money and status? What if you decided to prioritise disposable time over disposable income: *doing* things rather than *having* things? Until a few years ago, in the face of rampant Western capitalism, the shoots of the greener, co-operative sharing economy seemed unlikely to flourish – but look at how the world of work has changed. Self-expression does not have to mean poverty; freedom does not have to mean failure. You can be your own boss; you can find work which interests you *and* pays the bills. It's entirely within your control to rethink your priorities.

Professor John Ashton, president of the UK Faculty of Public Health, believes that how we work affects our health, not just our daily routine. He calls for a replacement of the five-day working week with a four-day model, 'so that people can enjoy their lives, have more time with their families, and maybe reduce high blood pressure'.

His four-day model is unlikely to take off in UK offices anytime soon, but the concept is important. It's driven by the primal belief that our well-being, both mental and physical, matters more than our salary, job title or quantifiable output. Having a rewarding career does not rule out having a happy personal life. We can be responsible workers *and* healthy individuals.

Taking a primal approach to your work means aiming for this balance of professional and personal; in essence, finding a balance between money and meaning. Working primally will take us in different directions: whether practical or artistic or scientific, collaborative or solitary, local or global; we all find fulfilment in our own way. Pursuing this primal work-life blend may well involve periods of uncertainty and self-doubt; it will probably entail compromise and determination. But it will be worth it, because when you find work that you love, you won't mind when it unbalances your life.

Chapter 6
Primal Eating

It's one of the mysteries of the modern age: why is healthy food so expensive and unhealthy food so cheap? Why does natural, unprocessed food cost more than heavily processed food? Freshness and flavour, sunshine and good soil, delicate herbs and subtle spices – surely these are the ingredients of delicious food, rather than artificial additives and preservatives that get consumers addicted and extend shelf life. If you've travelled to India, the Caribbean or the Mediterranean, if you've dug vegetables from an allotment or picked fruit in an orchard, you'll know that primal eating is a joy and a privilege.

From small cafés and posh delis to huge supermarkets, fresh fruit, salads, unsalted nuts and raw, natural ingredients are consistently more expensive than their calorific equivalents of pizzas, burgers, sausage rolls, doughnuts, muffins and fizzy drinks.

Healthy food is priced up, and junk food is at rock-bottom prices. Organic muesli costs three times the price of sugary breakfast cereals; a small punnet of raspberries or blueberries costs four times as much as a giant-sized bar of chocolate. Is it any wonder that public health is fraught with socio-economic issues? How are we all supposed to eat super-healthy goji berries, almond milk, chia seeds and avocados when they cost a bomb?

Instead of being able to buy natural, nutritious food, financial pressures on family budgets mean that many are filling up on high-sugar, high-salt, over-processed food substitutes. And yet, eating plentiful, pleasurable food shouldn't have to be this complicated or expensive. Food comes from the earth beneath our feet. Eating well is one of the most important parts of the primal journey.

Primal Appetite

In a world which is increasingly mixed-up about eating, it's important to work out what food is and why it matters. Hunger is the most primal of all needs. Humans and animals are instinctively programmed to seek out sustenance, whether that's a newborn baby blindly rooting for its mother's nipple, a caveman pursuing wild game or even crash survivors resorting to cannibalism in order to stay alive. We are programmed for life, and life requires food.

In the 1940s, the psychologist Abraham Maslow designed a pyramid ranking different human needs on different layers. His 'Hierarchy of Needs' (see below) demonstrates how our needs motivate our behaviour: until humans have fulfilled their basic survival requirements – for food, water, shelter and warmth – at the base of the pyramid, they cannot move up the layers to fulfil any of the more complex needs at the top.

Hunger and thirst matter more than anything else. Love, friendship and self-expression are important too, but Maslow's pyramid is a reminder that without the basic fuel which drives all life, those higher-order needs cannot be reached. You're unlikely to have the creative energy to compose love sonnets if you haven't eaten for a week.

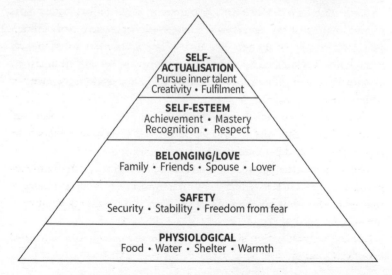

The pyramid isn't rocket science; in fact, it seems pretty obvious. Yet we still struggle with this basic understanding of the role of food. We know that moderation is key and balance is best but somehow the message gets scrambled along the way. From excess to deprivation, yo-yo dieting to bingeing, obesity to anorexia and everything in between, society is reaching crisis point. According to Diabetes UK, the number of people with diabetes is up 60 per cent in the last decade; around 90 per cent of these have type 2 diabetes (closely associated with obesity). It's not just a British problem: according to the International Diabetes Federation, more than 371 million people across the globe have diabetes. This figure is predicted to rise to over 550 million by 2030.

Is it any wonder that we've become so confused about food? Here in the affluent West, we're surrounded by temptations to top up on calories in every area of daily life: at train stations and at airports, on the high street, in hospital vending machines, at the gym, the petrol station and the cinema, and in every café and juice bar.

If all these inviting calories weren't bad enough, we're bombarded with scaremongering health warnings and general overload of contradictory nutritional information. How do we make sense of it all? Does fat make us fat or is it healthy to follow a low-carb, high-fat regime? Should we eat more protein or less? Should we steer clear of the sugar in fruit? And what about eggs and cholesterol? What's the right balance of omega-3, 6 and 9? Should we fast for two days a week and eat for five, or is it the other way around? Will ingesting clay really purify our insides? Should we be eating like werewolves or like cavemen?

It's hard not to be confused by all this nutritional noise and misinformation, and the endless tips and tricks offered up as shortcuts to weight loss and perfect health.

This is where the primal mindset comes in. Eating primally means going back to basics: exploring your personal tastes, finding a balance that works for your body and your lifestyle, and redefining what food means to you.

Remember that eating should be a pleasure as well as a source of fuel. Guilt and anxiety have no place on your plate.

Each to Their Own

Above all, it's essential to eat food that makes *you* feel good. It's no good following regimes which are said to be healthy but make you feel rotten. We all have different eating habits, taste buds, metabolic and digestive systems.

Have the confidence to decide what you need. If certain foods leave you feeling bloated or sleepy, irritable or instantly hungry again, they're not right for you. If carbs give you energy, enjoy them; if protein makes you feel strong, go for it. Don't cut out caffeine if that morning espresso is one of your daily pleasures; don't eliminate dairy if you really love cheese. Life is for living, after all.

Experiment with flavours and get to know your own digestive system: just because you're born in the UK, it doesn't mean you can't borrow from Japanese, Icelandic or Mediterranean eating habits. At some point, you have to make the choice to end the anxiety and just eat what works for you, within reason. This will be food which makes your body feel nourished, which doesn't make you gain or lose too much weight, which you can afford, which doesn't wreck the environment and which tastes good.

Virtue vs Vice?

Labelling foods as sinful or naughty only makes them seem more desirable: like any forbidden pleasure, the more you deprive yourself, the more you crave the illicit substance. However, it can be helpful to have a rough idea of how healthy and not-so-healthy foods will fit into your diet. Without laying down food 'rules', I'd advocate a 90/10 balance: aiming to eat really well 90 per cent of the time, and allowing yourself indulgences in the remaining 10 per cent. Hopefully, if you're enjoying the good 'healthy' stuff, this won't feel like deprivation, because you're relishing all the food you eat, all the time. This tactic also means you'll avoid the binge-starve-crave cycle created by cutting out entire food groups, or attempting drastic fasting regimes.

A Word About Oils

We often hear about the health benefits of eating more like our European neighbours, especially their regular consumption of olive oil. Most of us have at least one bottle of 'extra virgin' in the kitchen.

But olive is not the only oil! The food writers and TV cooks Hugh Fearnley-Whittingstall and Nigella Lawson are passionate advocates of cold-pressed rapeseed oil. Nigella in particular extols its nutty flavours and golden hues. Rapeseed is versatile and tasty; you can use it instead of olive oil for most recipes, as a salad dressing, or even spread it on toast instead of butter.

Home-grown British rapeseed oil is also less expensive and more environmentally friendly, so you can feel virtuous as well as healthy. The UK's production of rapeseed oil has risen from a few thousand tonnes in the 1970s to a couple of million today, almost doubling in the past decade alone.

In the kitchen (as in the bathroom) coconut oil is invaluable. It's a versatile sweetener and works well as a binder. Add it to cakes, raw baking, cookies, smoothies and porridge. With its high smoke point, coconut oil is also useful in savoury cooking – try it in place of olive oil in stir-fries or when roasting vegetables. Coconut milk, coconut yogurt, coconut juice and coconut ice cream are increasingly popular alternatives to dairy and a healthy way to cut down on refined sugars. Coconut creates the same smooth texture and tastes just as creamy. A large tub of high-quality coconut oil costs between £5 and £10 and lasts for ages: go for the raw, unrefined, organic version available in supermarkets and health food shops. It is solid at room temperature and turns to liquid when heated. NB do keep your bathroom and kitchen supplies separate – you don't want grated carrot in your hair mask or eyelashes in your stir-fry.

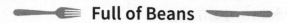 Full of Beans

Sometimes even vegetarians fancy a burger! This one is substantial, packed with nutritious ingredients and requires no cooking at all.

Recipe makes 8 burgers (they keep well in the fridge):

400 g tin kidney beans, drained
400 g tin black beans, drained
½ tsp ground cumin
2 tbsp chipotle paste
4 spring onions, trimmed and chopped
Small bunch coriander, chopped
150 g jar of roasted red peppers, drained
75 g crispy fried onions, crushed
250 g pack cooked quinoa
100 g cherry tomatoes
Pinch of sugar
8 burger buns
2 little gem lettuces, leaves separated

In a food processor, blend the kidney beans and black beans, cumin, chipotle paste, spring onions, half the coriander and 50 g red peppers into a thick, coarse puree.

Tip into a large mixing bowl and stir through the rest of the coriander, cooked quinoa and 25 g of fried onions. Season to taste. Form the mixture into eight roughly similar-sized burgers. Transfer onto a plate, cover and chill for around 20 minutes to firm up.

Chop the cherry tomatoes and remaining red peppers. Toss in a bowl with the sugar, and season.

Split and toast the burger buns. Press the remaining fried onions onto the burgers. Serve in the buns garnished with the red peppers and cherry tomato mixture, and gem lettuce.

Magic Mushrooms

What could be more natural than coming across a crop of fresh, white, just-blooming mushrooms, still damp from the dew? The humble fungi are packed-full of nutritional goodness and healing properties. They're also plentiful and delicious, and a great replacement for meat in vegetarian and vegan risottos, curries and stir-fries.

For centuries mushrooms have been used in traditional Chinese medicine to alleviate everything from hay fever to high blood pressure. They're also an essential component of modern pharmaceuticals, from statins for cholesterol to antibiotics like penicillin. An excellent source of B vitamins, vitamin D, iron and zinc, mushrooms are good for the immune system, for reducing inflammation and for boosting energy. Mushrooms are used in nutritional supplements, herbal teas and even super-healthy chocolate. They increasingly feature in exclusive cosmetics and beauty products, such as skin serums, cleansers, clay masks and even fragrances.

There are around 10,000 species of fungi scientifically identified, but this is only a fraction of what's out there. Some mycologists suspect there could be as many as ten million species in the world. You'll know about shiitake, portobello and button mushrooms; here are a few others to look out for.

- **Chaga mushrooms.** Chagas are said to contain more antioxidants than any other food in the world. With notes of caramel and vanilla, they are tasty, too – try wild chaga tea.

- **Reishi mushrooms.** Reishi are anti-inflammatory and help to balance overactive stress hormones. You can take reishi capsules, or drink it as a relaxing bedtime tea.

- **Cordyceps mushrooms.** Cordyceps provide a natural energy boost by increasing levels of ATP, a compound used by the body to store and transport energy in cells. Cordyceps chocolate provides a virtuous alternative when you hit that afternoon slump.

How to Shop

Wild mushrooms, still damp from the dew, may be primal – but unfortunately most of us have to procure our food in less poetic environments. In an ideal world we'd pick all our vegetables from the allotment and all our fruit from the orchard... But in the real world we're far more likely to be somewhere on the high street.

We do still have a choice about how and where we buy our food. Consumer patterns and spending habits are very individual: maybe you shop online and have your groceries delivered by one of the big four supermarkets; perhaps you consciously prefer to shop locally and support your neighbourhood greengrocer, butcher or baker. Time and financial pressures are increasing all the time, as well as the multitude of health warnings and fads, claims and counter-claims about what is best for you and the planet.

Likewise, whether or not you choose to buy organic is up to you. While there is no doubt that organic produce carries a price premium and is not affordable for everyone, there are many health and environmental concerns to be weighed up. Many consumers choose organic versions of certain products, for example fruit and vegetables, which otherwise come into closest contact with potentially harmful fertilisers or chemicals.

Supplements

From vitamin-infused water to Adriatic krill, to black rice bran and wheatgrass shots, the range of superfood supplements, powders and potions is bewildering. Promising to cure everything, including skin complaints, digestive problems, fatigue and depression – even to reverse ageing – it's wise to take most of these miracle products with a hefty dose of scepticism.

There is no harm in taking a good quality multi-vitamin supplement. Some specific supplements are known to carry genuine benefits: vitamin D can be helpful in winter, for example, and iron if you're anaemic (fairly common among women of childbearing age). Some people swear by a short course of echinacea during the cold and flu season. And of course some supplements are considered essential: for example, folic acid before and during pregnancy, or vitamin K for newborn babies.

However, it's generally considered healthier to get your nutrients from food, in their natural 'bioavailable' form, rather than as pills. Some miracle supplements are not only a waste of money, but they can even be unsafe. Unlike other medicines, the lucrative market of vitamins and nutritional supplements is barely regulated in the UK. Producers frequently make unsubstantiated claims, with fraudulent labelling promising all sorts of health benefits.

For example, vitamin E and beta-carotene have been scientifically proven to be useless – even harmful – when taken in isolation (*Annals of Internal Medicine*, 2014). It's thought that vitamin C or zinc may cause nausea, diarrhoea and stomach cramps. Too much selenium can lead to hair loss, gastrointestinal upset, fatigue and mild nerve damage.

It's important not to exceed the recommended daily dose of any vitamins or mineral. Professor Marion Nestle argues against the over-reliance on supplements: 'It takes the nutrient out of the context of the food, the food out of the context of the diet, and the diet out of the context of the lifestyle.'

Of course, our cave-dwelling ancestors didn't have the option of taking multi-vitamins, but that doesn't mean they don't have their place. Specific supplementation can be essential if you have a particular deficiency, or during periods of stress or depression. Always consult your doctor if you're feeling depleted or otherwise unwell. The best advice is to stay primal with your body, keeping in touch with how you're feeling and functioning. When you're tuned into your body's physical and emotional messages, it will be easier to pick up on problems.

The White Stuff

Milk is a conundrum in more ways than one. In the form of breast milk, it's often a baby's earliest sustenance. The miracle of a mother's milk is deeply primal: it protects the baby from infections and diseases, is available on demand, and builds a strong emotional and physical bond between mother and child. Milk is a rich source of calcium, and considered to be essential for building healthy bones and teeth in infancy. The importance of milk in childhood continues long after weaning: many of us will remember the little glass bottles or cartons of milk we were given as schoolchildren at break-time.

But is it all that primal? The milk we drink as children and adults is very different to that early mother's milk. Vegans do not consume dairy in any form, citing the unnatural conditions behind the milk production industry. They disapprove of the fact that female cows are repeatedly artificially inseminated, then separated from their calves after birth and pumped full of hormones to keep them in more or less constant lactation.

When compared to sugar-laden fizzy drinks, milk does still seem like a primal, natural option. As well as calcium, it's a rich source of magnesium, potassium, selenium, zinc, vitamins A, B6, B12, and D, and protein. Millions of gallons are consumed every day – on cereal, in coffee and in tea – and it's a staple ingredient in everything from cheese to yogurt to milkshakes to many cakes. However, as there are so many alternatives available these days, such as coconut yogurt, almond milk and soya-based cheeses, dairy-based foods are no longer essential.

Whether or not you're vegan, there are moral questions around the consumption of milk. Due to a global increase in milk production and a slump in demand, the UK dairy industry is in crisis, with an average of one or two farms closing every day. In recent years milk has become a major pawn in the retailers' price war: most of the big supermarkets now sell 4 pints of milk for less than £1. In other words, it costs the farmer more to produce the milk than it actually earns. Milk is now cheaper than bottled water.

Just as we choose how we eat and what we're prepared to spend, so milk is an individual choice. Is drinking milk from cows primal or simply unnatural and exploitative? Is it even good for us? For me, buying organic milk helps to address some, if not all, of the health and ethical issues. It costs 10 or 20 pence extra per pint, but it feels fairer to the cattle and farmers, and I notice the difference in taste. Surely, we should be prepared to pay at least the cost price for our own health and the welfare of the animals that produce these valuable nutrients?

To Eat or To Drink?

As a rule, it's better to eat, rather than drink, your fruit. Can you imagine cavemen or cavewomen pressing their berries, drinking the juice and then *discarding* the flesh? Primal eating is all about working with ingredients in their most natural form.

Nutritionists generally concur that we should eat rather than drink our fruit and vegetables. Numerous studies have shown that drinking sugary fruit juice can be as damaging to health as fizzy drinks. As just one example of this, the rise in blood-sugar level which occurs after drinking apple juice is much higher than after eating an apple.

The reason is simple: juicing destroys the important insoluble fibre in fruit, so the body is bombarded with high levels of the natural sugar, fructose. The liver becomes overwhelmed with it and converts it to liver fat, increasing the likelihood of insulin resistance, diabetes and heart disease. The chief nutritionist at Public Health England, Dr Alison Tedstone explains that juicing 'significantly increases your free sugar intake... which is the same as added sugar in processed food'. Drinking acidic juices also strips tooth enamel and leads to dental decay.

There's also the fact that juicing your fruit makes it easy to over-consume. It's well-known that drinking calories do not register in the same way as eating them. When was the last time you ate four apples, a banana and a handful of strawberries all in one go? Yet when juiced, this kind of quantity of fresh fruit is easy to ingest, giving you around 20 teaspoons of sugar in a single hit (minus the healthy fibre which slows down digestion and satiates in whole fruit).

While there is no doubt that fruit does contain fructose, it is in its most natural form. To me, anything that grows on trees or bushes, ripens in the sunshine, and is so clearly bursting with flavour, colour and vitamins is always going to be a healthier option than soft drinks or confectionary. However, it's important that we take the overall levels of fructose into account in our daily diets. This means that, wherever you can, it's best to eat your fruit and veg whole, raw or lightly steamed.

If you really can't give up your daily juice, a home-made smoothie can still offer health benefits that processed junk food cannot, as we'll see. If you're concerned and want to limit your intake of natural sugars, keep an eye out for these high and low fructose fruit and vegetables.

Guide to high and low fructose	
Low fructose fruit	grapefruit, melon, oranges, raspberries, strawberries
High fructose fruit	banana, blueberries, grapes, kiwi
Low fructose vegetables	spinach, watercress, cucumber, green beans, kale

Juices and Smoothies

A nutritionist colleague pointed out that some yogurt frappuccinos contain over 400 calories and up to 20 grams of fat: 'Just because it contains the words strawberry, mango or passion fruit doesn't make it one of your five a day – and it doesn't make it healthy! These yogurty, creamy, sugary beverages are a long way from the original fruit, and offer little in the way of vitamins or minerals. Just because you're drinking it in a coffee chain doesn't make it a drink – this is a small meal! Fine as an occasional treat, but *not* every day with your morning coffee.'

But there is no avoiding the great juicing movement. Instagram is awash with the green juices and breakfast smoothies of the rich and the beautiful: top models, actresses and fashionistas slurping back their kale, spirulina and spinach like there's no tomorrow. Juicing gurus claim to cure everything from asthma to psoriasis, infertility to cancer, and their books and DVDs sell in their millions.

Lakeland saw a barely believable 4,000 per cent rise in juicers bought last year, and Vitamix have tripled their sales over the past five years. Ever more advanced, gleaming, space-age gadgets for pulping cold-pressing and blending fill the shops. (Remember when we used to squeeze an orange by hand, with those plastic ridged egg-shaped things on top of a glass?)

However, there are juices and then there are *juices*. Shop-bought concoctions, including those which claim to be 100 per cent natural or have cutesy names (and cutesy marketing messages on the side about being free of nasties), are usually heat-treated or pasteurised. This process destroys a large proportion of the vitamins and minerals. Crucially, it also destroys the enzyme activity, which is the life force of the plant.

As for shop-bought smoothies, the proportion of fresh ingredients is often negligible. The base juice is often from concentrate or pasteurised juice, and some contain more sugar-loaded fat-free yogurt than actual fruit. Heat-treated, bottled smoothies can sit in a supermarket chiller for over a week. Check the side of the bottle: do you recognise all the ingredients or do you see stabilisers, emulsifiers and other artificial extras?

Golden Oldies

If you're happy with simple (old-style) juices, here are three of the scientifically proven-best!

Beetroot: ideal before exercise. A recent study in the American Journal of Physiology found that that drinking beetroot juice can help you to work out for longer; it also assists your heart in supplying oxygen to muscles more effectively.

Watermelon: ideal after exercise. Spanish scientists have discovered that watermelon juice can reduce muscle soreness after a workout and also recovery heart rate.

Pear: ideal for a hangover. Australian researchers claim that a cup of pear juice before an alcoholic night on the tiles can lead to fewer hangover symptoms, including headache and nausea.

Paying Over the Odds

These drinks often come with a hefty price tag, especially in the more exclusive juice cafés and vitality bars. (Hint: there will be lots of beautiful people in workout gear while others will be wearing sunglasses and having breakfast meetings.) I recently had brunch with a naturopath friend at his favourite organic juicery in central London. Our cold-pressed green juices cost nearly £10 a glass.

To save you the money, we drank 'Green Incredibles', containing apple, celery, lemon, banana, kale, fresh coconut, aloe vera, wild Irish moss and superfoody greens powders... They did taste 'incredible', but think how much fresh fruit and vegetables (and maybe even Irish moss) you could have bought for that price!

Prices for bespoke, home-delivery juice cleanses are even more staggering. A range of companies offer detoxifying, energising, radiance bottles of raw juice three-day cleanses for anything from £200–£400. For all the cashew milk, coconut butter, Himalayan sea salt and low-alkaline ingredients, it still seems like a lot of money to starve yourself for three days.

Do-It-Yourself

The best way to ensure that your juices or smoothies contain all the good stuff, and none of the unnecessary additions, is to make them yourself. For the equivalent of that single expensive juice I described before, you can buy a basketful of fresh produce. Blitzing up a load of fruit as a quick breakfast on the run makes a great start to the day, and boosts your intake of vitamins and minerals. It's also a fantastic way to use up the contents of your fruit bowl and fridge if things are reaching the end of their natural life or if you're going away (because living primally means never wasting food). Adding vegetables to your juice is also tasty and nutritious.

Moreover, fresh juices and smoothies are a cunning way to get children to consume a good daily portion of vegetables. Even the most veg-phobic child won't detect carrot, spinach or broccoli thrown into their fruit juice!

Another good reason to avoid shop-bought juices, and instead make your own, is that your body will register the process of being fed. Our primal ancestors worked hard for every calorie: whether it was foraging for nuts, picking berries or hunting animals. Whatever they ate, they had earned – and that's something we've lost in the convenience food culture. No matter how healthy our chosen café may be, handing over a tenner for your lunchtime wrap and smoothie is not the same as preparing it yourself. Eating primally involves being mindful about your food: touching the ingredients, smelling the flavours and savouring the results.

This won't always mean cooking from scratch – for most of us, that's impossible during the working day. However, there are genuine benefits to preparing your fruit for juicing, even if it's just peeling a banana, chopping an apple, and throwing a few raspberries and ice cubes on top. You're likely to consume more of the whole fruit, and to drink it when it's absolutely fresh, with all the nutrients at their best. Blitzing it up and pouring it out into a tall glass is far more satisfying than buying an overpriced plastic bottle (more pollution) from a whirring industrial fridge. You could whizz up a batch at breakfast and decant it into a bottle or flask to take into the office with you, just as you would with healthy dinner leftovers for your work lunch.

Juicers, Blenders and Smoothie Makers

Blenders just blend (!) while juicers extract the juice from the actual pulp. It's a matter of taste: if you dislike pulp in your drink, you'd be better go for a juicer; I love having the whole fruit in there, although it can involve more preparation, such as chopping and deseeding of apple and pears, for example. Alternatively, you can use a combination of techniques: juicing the pineapple, for example and then adding to berries in the blender. As for smoothie makers, some nutritionists say that these are just blenders with a tap.

These days you can spend as much or as little as you want. At the premium end of the range are the all-singing, all-dancing, added horsepower juicers, some costing thousands of pounds. They extract maximum nutrition from raw food, cold-press, remove pulp, conserve precious fruit enzymes, pulverise skins and seeds, and even make coulis and heat soups. Cold-pressing is a method of juicing which ensures that no heat is used in the process. It's a hydraulic press which squashes the fruit and vegetables. As there is no heat, none of the nutrients are destroyed or wasted.

Slightly less glitzy are the standard centrifugal juicers, which are reliable, popular and affordable.

Or you can still just go for the basic food processor/blender, ideal for tight budgets. In my early forays into juicing I started out using a handheld soup blender. I experienced some difficulties (OK, breaks) with ice cubes or hard fruits, but they work fine for soft fruits, frozen fruits and avocados. Hint: this can get messy – use a bowl with tall sides!

An essential aspect of going primal is using and reusing what we already have, rather than mindlessly buying and discarding – especially in the case of bulky plastic appliances. If you're one of those people who have a lot of unused kitchen gadgets (and most of us do), I'd humbly suggest that you look in your cupboards first. You probably already own a blender or food processor which will be more than capable of making smoothies. Maybe use that a few times to see if it's a habit you're going to stick with – or try out a friend's juicer. There's nothing worse than adding to the pile of unused kitchen/exercise equipment/mobiles/chargers we all accumulate.

Food Waste

It's not only kitchen gadgets that we buy and waste, but food too. Have you ever found yourself standing in front of the fruit bowl, wondering why some pears remain rock-hard for weeks? How did that banana go from too-green to too-ripe in the blink of an eye?

These, and many other kitchen mysteries, mean that we often waste perfectly good food. Eating primally means thinking creatively about the produce you buy and doing everything you can to cut out waste. (The banana bread recipe on page 148, for example, will eliminate all banana waste for evermore.) Food and water are among the Earth's most precious resources; everything we harvest is a valuable source of energy. When you think carefully about what you buy and consume, and when you're determined not to throw anything away, it becomes easy, almost automatic, to eat more primally and less wastefully.

It's a sad fact that the UK is the most wasteful nation in Europe. British households throw out an average 6 kg of food per week, which amounts to between 7 and 8 million tonnes of food a year, more than half of which is perfectly safe and edible. When you include the food wasted by manufacturers, retailers and restaurants, that figure rises to around 18–20 million tonnes wasted annually in the UK. Between 20–40 per cent of edible fruit and vegetables are rejected before they reach the shops because of cosmetic standards: that knobbly carrot which doesn't conform to criteria of straight-ness or orange-ness, for example, or a slightly wonky courgette.

The French are taking a robust attitude to the issue of food waste with a new law from 2016 which legally obliges supermarkets to donate their unsold food to charity. The law also forces restaurants to provide containers for customers to take uneaten food home with them (amusingly called '*le doggy bag*' or '*la box anti-gaspi*').

The French are not the only ones: the brilliant website www. neighbourly.com, which promotes co-operation within communities, has been pioneering food donation on a nationwide scale. They put big supermarkets and food outlets in touch with local charities and community projects that can use food, sometimes with slightly damaged packaging but still safely within date.

Food scientists at the University of the West of England believe that extending 'sell by' dates on fresh produce could make a huge difference: 'One extra day of life for fresh produce will reduce waste, could save millions and help resolve global hunger.' When you think about everyday items like cherry tomatoes, potatoes and carrots – all safe and edible beyond the 'sell by' date – it becomes clear what a huge amount of waste such a simple strategy could prevent.

Some eco-friendly entrepreneurs have started thinking about the problem of food waste. Several apps aimed at helping people share the contents of their fridge with neighbours, rather than throwing food away, have been launched. They allow individuals, small shops and cafés to post pictures of food, drink and other groceries they don't need, and then arrange to collect from each other. It's a creative, positive way to avoid waste when you're going on holiday, moving house or simply can't use up what you have in the fridge or fruit bowl.

It's estimated that if we reduced global food waste by a quarter, there would be enough food to feed the entire world. This wasted food could not only have fed hungry people, but its production also generates greenhouse gas emissions and consumes vast quantities of water – all for nothing.

Why *are* we wasting so much food? Mostly, it's due to a lack of understanding: a 2013 study found that that 90 per cent of Americans were confused by the different dates and warnings on food packages (Natural Resources Defense Council and Harvard Law School). Most of us glance at 'sell by', 'best before' and 'use by' dates and assume they mean the same thing. However, this isn't the case. Here's what they really mean.

✓ **Sell by** date is when the maker advises the store to remove the product from its shelves.

✓ **Best before** date is when the maker believes the product will reach the end of its peak quality. It doesn't mean that the food isn't safe after that.

✓ **Use by** date is the last date by which the manufacturer says the product should be used.

They may look official, but most dates are merely suggestions by the manufacturer, as guidance on how long to display the product and when it's at its best quality. They are not necessarily safety dates.

Many foods can be safely and enjoyably consumed well after their designated dates, provided that adequate care is taken during storage.

Milk, for example, will last in the fridge a good five to seven days after its marked expiry date.

Eggs are usually fine for an additional three to four weeks.

Dried pasta will last for a couple of years beyond its best before date.

Tinned tuna is fine for up to five years.

Of course, it's sensible to discard milk which smells or tastes 'off'. The same goes for fish and meat that are past their use by date, or anything obviously spoiled, although many people scrape mould off cheese and safely eat it! But we live in an age of refrigeration and freezing, and we can preserve and consume food more safely than our ancestors – even our parents and grandparents – could have dreamed of. Taking a primal approach to food waste is simple: it means thinking about food before we buy it, and using it before it goes off.

Juice-fasts and Liquid-only Diets

Many people go on liquid-only diets in order to lose a lot of weight in a short space of time. Juice-fasts, i.e. fasting for prolonged periods without solid food, are really not recommended. For all the claims surrounding this type of fasting (especially around weight loss) there is no objective scientific evidence for it. Most experts would argue the opposite: it encourages the kind of yo-yo cycle of craving and bingeing which is the enemy of healthy, long-term weight management. Additionally, going without solid food for days can be downright dangerous, causing dizziness, nausea and hypoglycaemia.

Even Michael Moseley, the doctor who invented the 5:2 fasting diet, is critical of juicing fasts: 'You need protein to fill you up. Unless you have adequate amounts of it, within 24 hours your body starts to cannibalise itself and get protein from your muscles. A juice diet is zero protein so you will lose a small amount of fat and a large amount of muscle. And if you lose muscle your metabolic rate will slow down.'

Clearly, juice-fasts are not the answer to long-term sustained weight loss, and neither are they a solution to emotional or overeating, or other problematic relationships with food. Fasting may be primal in the strictest sense, as cavemen would sometimes have gone without food through necessity, but modern forms of fasting often lead to unhealthy cycles of crash-dieting and bingeing.

Detoxing?

As for detoxing, it's simply not necessary. Despite all the marketing hype about hidden toxins and the need to purify, we have powerful systems inside our bodies: our liver, kidneys, bladder and bowels. They are designed to process our food and eliminate waste products

– and unless we're ill or seriously overdoing it, they carry out their function adequately. Apart from the liver, which clearly benefits from alcohol-free regeneration, the rest of our organs don't actually need detoxification.

Detoxing is a relatively recent obsession. Only a few decades ago, perfectly healthy people would have looked at you blankly if you'd suggested 'going on a detox'. Terms such as 'low-carbing' and 'eating clean' had not been invented, and the notion of 'flushing out toxins' was non-existent. Previous generations ate well, with a good balance of food groups, even though their diets were not organic, macrobiotic or biodynamic. What's more, they knew nothing of antioxidants, and they never went on detox diets!

> Here's what the experts say about detoxing and juice-fasting:
>
> **Russell Bateman, fitness guru:** 'Doing a detox involving fluids only makes almost no difference to the chemical build-up in our bodies. It can take 6–10 years of zero exposure to get rid of half the amount of fat soluble chemicals in our body. Zero exposure these days is impossible! Count the chemicals in your foods, buy high quality produce and ditch the fads.'
>
> **Ian Marber, nutritionist and author:** 'You don't need to try to "detox" any more than you need to try to breathe. It happens anyway.'
>
> **Zoë Harcombe, obesity researcher:** 'Detoxing is a nonsense term; it's not a physiological thing. You can give your liver a bit of a rest by having a few days off alcohol, not smoking, not eating processed food, but it's detoxifying all the time. The idea that giving it juice will help is nonsense.'

Detoxing may be unnecessary, but there's nothing wrong with giving your body a spring clean.

Eat more fresh foods in their natural, unprocessed state.

- Add plenty of vegetables to every meal, raw or lightly steamed, and as snacks.

- Cut down on salt, sugar and artificial ingredients.

- Avoid polluted traffic-choked roads.

- Go somewhere green and breathe in the amazing fresh air!

- And if you've had a period of heavy drinking, say during the festive season, or you've been eating a lot of rich or processed food, increasing your fruit and veg intake is a great idea.

Spring Clean Juice

This juice is packed with nutrients: make it at home and drink it fresh. **Blend:** 2 apples, 1 carrot, 1 slice lemon with rind, ¼ yellow pepper, 1 inch slice of cucumber, 1/4 piece of celery, 1 inch broccoli stem, 1 inch slice raw beetroot and ice.

Contains: vitamins B1, B2, B3, B5 B6, C, E and K, calcium, iron, magnesium, pectin, boron, beta-carotene, potassium, phosphorus, selenium, folic acid, riboflavin, and phytonutrients.

Benefits? Packed with anti-cancer phytonutrients and also beta-carotene to strengthen the immune system and mop up free radicals. Celery reduces acidity and flushes out excess carbon dioxide. Beetroot cleans the bloodstream and builds blood, and cleanses the liver and kidneys.

Salad Smoothie

Blend: 2 apples, ½ stick of celery, 1 inch chunk of cucumber, 1 big handful of spinach, 1 small handful watercress, ½ ripe avocado and 4 ice cubes. Juice the apples, cucumber, celery, spinach and watercress, and then blend this juice with the flesh of the avocado and ice.

Contains: Avocados are considered pretty much 'complete' foods, containing essential fats, natural sugars, amino acids, vitamins, minerals and enzymes. Spinach contains chlorophyll, beta-carotene, folic acid, iron, choline, and vitamins A, C and E.

Great Gut Food

Vegetables are much lower in sugar than fruit, but here too the juicing-versus-eating debate is relevant. The fibre contained in the whole vegetable helps to keep your gut bacteria healthy, and this is lost when the vegetable is juiced.

There are around 100 trillion bacteria in your gut. They are essential for good digestion: absorbing micronutrients, processing vitamins and formulating enzymes. They also play a key role in fighting obesity, type 2 diabetes, heart disease, autoimmune disease and even certain forms of cancer. These microbes thrive on colourful plant-based foods. The more diversity you have in your gut-friendly bacteria, the healthier and more resilient your intestines and immune system.

Bacteria in the colon need a specific type of fibre called fructans, a form of prebiotic. They also need cellulose: an insoluble fibre which promotes good gut microbes. The parts of the vegetable that we tend to throw out are high in cellulose: the chewy stalks of broccoli, the fibrous tops of leeks, carrot peelings or the bottoms of asparagus. Heat breaks down fibre, so don't overcook: consider using shavings of broccoli stems, raw asparagus or artichokes in salads, or quickly grill or stir-fry whole leeks: delicious in oil! Introduce more of this gut-friendly fibre into your diet gradually, in order to avoid bloating or gas.

Good for Guts...

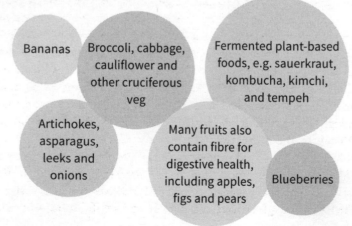

Bananas

Broccoli, cabbage, cauliflower and other cruciferous veg

Fermented plant-based foods, e.g. sauerkraut, kombucha, kimchi, and tempeh

Artichokes, asparagus, leeks and onions

Many fruits also contain fibre for digestive health, including apples, figs and pears

Blueberries

Hidden Nasties

It's no secret that governments and consumers are increasingly concerned about the growing levels of obesity in populations across the world, from India to America to Europe. Global food manufacturers have spent billions developing that perfect ratio of salt, sugar and fat: that moreish balance which keeps us wanting more, more, more – never satiated or properly nourished, but always reaching for the next bag of crisps or fizzy drink. We gorge on empty calories which give us a massive sugar rush and then crash – always leaving us craving more. Interestingly, the least processed foods have been found to be the least addictive, including salmon, beans, broccoli and apples.

Scientific research has helped to shed light on why we crave the unhealthiest foods. In studies, chocolate is routinely rated as the number one craving, closely followed by other processed foods, including pizza, ice cream, crisps, cake and biscuits. Unsurprisingly, the most craved foods have the highest levels of added fat or refined carbohydrates, such as white flour and sugar. These products stimulate the brain's pleasure centre, making you feel good, and making you want more, more, more. Alarmingly, studies on laboratory rats have shown sugar to be more addictive than cocaine.

The excessive levels of sugar, salt and fat in our food are particularly shocking because they're hidden, or at least not in the places we expect them to be. Consumer tests have highlighted the worst offenders: a ready meal of sweet-and-sour chicken, for example, contains ten teaspoons of sugar (more than a bar of chocolate); a sandwich from a high-street fast-food chain contains the same amount of salt as nine bags of ready salted crisps; a cheddar ploughman's sandwich from a leading supermarket contains more than three-quarters of an adult woman's daily recommended saturated fat intake. It also contained very high levels of sugar: who would expect sugar in their cheese sarnie?

Obviously these are twenty-first-century – even 'first world' – problems. Modern food production has undoubtedly given us safer, fresher and healthier food than at any time in history, but it also presents us with this minefield of artificial additives and preservatives. We're lucky enough to have access to more plentiful food, and more varied flavours than ever before, but we also need to decide what level of 'hidden extras' we're comfortable with. As with other aspects of the primal lifestyle, this has to involve some degree of compromise. It's near-impossible to avoid all artificial ingredients, unless you adopt a raw-food diet, never buy convenience food and never eat out. Primal eating should be a guide, not a straitjacket, to encourage you to enjoy more of nature's freshest ingredients more often.

Herbs and Spices

The reason all those tempting 'convenience' foods are loaded up with sugar and salt is to give them flavour. Without artificial additives and preservatives, sugar and salt, especially when we're accustomed to high levels, food can taste bland and flavourless. Too often producers remove real flavour – usually fat – and replace it with fake flavour. Hence, so-called 'healthy' low-fat yogurts which contain more than five teaspoons of sugar in a single pot.

In fact, bland food is one of the main reasons that people cite for giving up on healthy eating plans: natural flavours are more delicate than the processed, overly sugary and salty food we're accustomed to. It takes a while for your taste buds to adjust.

The solution, of course, is simple: put the flavour back. And this is where herbs and spices come in. What could be more satisfying than adding herbs you've grown yourself (or even bought in a pot) to your cooking? What could be more positive and primal? At my parents' house in the South of France, my mother has planted a herb garden beside the kitchen door. When she's preparing lamb, she'll wander outside and snip some rosemary; for roasted vegetables she has dill, parsley and marjoram; for baby new potatoes there's fresh mint; for carrot soup there's coriander – and there's basil for everything else.

Even the least green-fingered among us can cultivate herbs. Try growing mint, thyme, rosemary, sage, chives or oregano. They're easy to look after and versatile in many different dishes. Scatter herbs into your omelette with joyful abandon: dill, tarragon and parsley taste wonderful with free-range eggs and goat's cheese.

As for spices, these can truly make a dish come alive. They have wide-ranging health benefits (and are virtually calorie-free); here are some of the most versatile.

Ginger: used widely in sweet and savoury dishes, ground dried ginger is great in baking. Fresh root ginger is used in curries and stir-fries, and also cold drinks. It is thought to be a miracle cure-all for everything from colds to nausea, inflammation to infertility.

Cumin: warm, pungent spice, used widely in Indian and North African cooking.

Coriander: warm, aromatic spice often paired with cumin, especially for spice rubs, used in Indian and Asian cooking. It's great in meat (and with carrots for delicious soup).

Garam masala: Indian mixture of ground spices of cumin, coriander, cardamom and black pepper. Buy it ready mixed or roasted and grind your own fresh spices.

Turmeric: bright, yellow spice with peppery, earthy flavour, widely used in Indian food. It improves symptoms of irritable bowel syndrome and aids digestion. It contains curcumin, which has powerful anti-inflammatory and healing qualities.

Fennel: little green seeds with sweet, aniseed-like flavour, great with chicken and fish, but also in breads.

Cloves: these dried flower buds have a strong, spicy flavour; can be used whole or ground in a variety of sweet and savoury dishes.

Cinnamon: can be used in stews and casseroles, or as a ground spice for baking and desserts. Thought to lower glucose and cholesterol levels, it is potentially beneficial in treating diabetes.

Nutmeg: my favourite! It adds a warm spiciness to milk, egg and creamy dishes, and also enhances spinach. Available as ground nutmeg, but even better when freshly grated: try it on your chai latte with vanilla pods or extract.

Purists will shudder, but you can buy easy spice mixes in supermarkets if you're not up for roasting and grinding your own. Some of the most useful include: Chinese five spices, harissa, Cajun seasoning or chilli flakes. Unusual combinations can taste amazing: a lentil stew with roast almonds and cinnamon, for example, or a sweet spice mix or cinnamon on hot porridge, in place of sugar, with honey and a splash of almond milk.

Avo-mania

Eating primally is all about fruit and vegetables, that much is clear. However, not all fruit and vegetables are exactly primal. Eating the delicious, and now deeply trendy, avocado is very good for your health… but it's not all that good for the planet.

Buzzfeed recently announced: 'The avocado is not an ingredient. It's a lifestyle.' Scooped, sliced, diced, mashed, smashed, whizzed, grilled or drizzled in oil, the avocado must be the first fruit to have its own hashtag. Supermodels, beauty editors, foodies and cookery writers rave about it; journalists love the pun-heavy headlines, from avo-mania to over-cado to avo-session to peak pear. Avocados are in our salads, sandwiches, smoothies and cakes, on our toast, even on our faces…

Now that we're all learning that eating fat does not make you fat, the knobbly fruit formerly known as the alligator pear is booming. The mania started in California and consumption has quintupled in the US over the past 15 years. UK supermarkets sales are up 33 per cent year on year, and the UK avocado market is now worth more than £50 million a year. Every year, American Super Bowl fans consume around 25,000 tons of avocado, in the form of guacamole, with their tortilla chips. Even Japan, China and South Korea have joined the global avo-mania.

Avocados are a potent source of essential fats, vitamin E and oleic (fatty) acids; they aid blood flow, protect heart and eye health, and have been called the 'complete food'. However, they are definitely not green. For example, the water footprint is one of the highest of any crop: estimates are as high as 100 litres (around 21 gallons) of water needed to produce a *single* avocado fruit. To put that in context, here are the water quantities needed to produce 1 pound of a range of fruit and vegetables (from www.treehugger.com).

Lettuce: 15 gallons
Tomatoes: 22 gallons
Cucumbers: 28 gallons
Potatoes: 30 gallons
Oranges: 55 gallons
Apples: 83 gallons
Mangoes: 190 gallons
Avocados: 220 gallons

The air miles involved in avocado consumption aren't much better. Most avocados are produced in Mexico, Peru, Chile, South Africa and Kenya, and flown around the world to cater for the all-year-round demand. Our craze for avocados has also a bad effect for the growers back home: the so-called 'green gold' is now such a valuable produce that indigenous farmers can no longer afford to eat them. The same thing has happened with quinoa. Until recently it was a staple grain for locals in Bolivia and Peru, but it has become so popular in Europe and the US that the locals end up exporting it and importing cheaper, refined (less healthy) food. From LA to Brooklyn to Clerkenwell, it seems that our appetite for these so-called 'superfoods' – think kelp, freekeh and goji berries – is insatiable.

Eating primally means eating fresh, yes, but it also means eating locally and seasonally. It entails thinking seriously about the planet. It doesn't mean depriving yourself – by all means, enjoy avocado as an occasional treat – but being aware of how far your food has come and what has gone into making it. Remember those towns in Chile where the avocado farmers used so much water that the local wells have run dry. And don't forget that astounding figure: the 100 litres of water it takes to grow a single fruit.

Alternative Superfoods

In reality, these so-called superfoods are no more *super* than plenty of other fresh, healthy produce: 'superfood' is an invented marketing term which has no basis in nutritional science. Those foreign juices, seeds or berries aren't magically anti-ageing, cancer-fighting or fertility-boosting, no matter how exotic they appear. Rather than paying over the odds for produce which has been flown halfway across the world, it's far better to go primal, support UK agriculture, and buy local and seasonal wherever possible. British potatoes or pears may not feel very exotic, but they're still rich in nutrients. See the Primal and Seasonal chapter for the full range of seasonal produce you can enjoy at different times of the year, at a far lower environmental cost.

The healthiest diet is fresh and varied, with a range of 'super' vitamins and minerals, nutrients and fibre. Eat the colours of the rainbow – orange carrots, red apples, purple broccoli, dark green kale, light green leeks, white cauliflower – and ignore the marketing hype. Above all, eat real food.

Allergies and Intolerances

Taking a primal approach to food also helps to avoid disordered or restrictive eating. The recent explosion of allergies and intolerances has been attributed, in part, to a collective uncertainty around the food industry. From the UK to Europe, the US to Australia, millions of people have decided, or have been persuaded, that they are allergic to certain foods, with the most commonly cited culprit being wheat. More than one in five Brits claim to have a food allergy or intolerance, an increase of 400 per cent in the past 20 years. However, research conducted by Portsmouth University has shown that of all those claiming to have an allergy or intolerance, only two per cent actually do. Similarly, in Europe the Allergen Bureau estimates that despite 30 per cent of adult Europeans claiming to experience adverse food reactions, only 3–5 per cent have been diagnosed with a genuine allergy.

Whole aisles in supermarkets are now dedicated to gluten-free products – even though, when questioned, most consumers don't actually know what gluten is or what it does. Far from being healthier, these products may be full of other 'nasties': gluten-free bread, biscuits and cereal, for example, often contain refined ingredients, such as additives, flavourings, stabilisers, added sugar and preservatives. And when you consider that these gluten-free products can cost up to five times as much as regular versions, they look a lot less tempting.

> 66 *When people have symptoms such as bloating, constipation, diarrhoea and food cravings, they often think they have an intolerance. In fact, this is way down the list of possibilities. True food intolerances are not common, and tests for them can be unreliable.* 99
> **Ian Marber, nutrition consultant**

Primal eating helps to counter this cycle of fearful food avoidance, because it focuses on quality, freshness and traceability. When we know where our food comes from, or when we've picked it ourselves, we don't need to eliminate specific foods or entire food groups.

Mankind has been harvesting wheat, milling flour, baking bread, milking cows, and churning butter and cheese for centuries. It therefore seems unlikely that these simple, primal ingredients should be triggering so many health problems. In fact, the most common genuine allergens are peanuts, shellfish, eggs and soya. These serious allergies can have fatal consequences, but are mercifully rare. And if anything in our modern lives should cause concern, shouldn't it be the new kids on the block: pollution, radio waves, parabens, industrial levels of artificial sweeteners and preservatives in food?

Instead of paying over the odds for these fake, refined, 'free-from' foods – worrying about non-existent dietary intolerances or avoiding wheat and gluten to lose weight – we might do better to opt for whole, natural, unrefined foods.

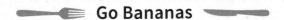 **Go Bananas**

I'm not much of a cook, but here's one of my few star turns! Banana bread is incredibly comforting, and this recipe is so simple that even

I can't mess it up. It's tasty enough to feel indulgent, but not too unhealthy. It's also an excellent way to counter food waste, using up any lurking bananas which are overly ripe.

Blend or mix by hand:

> 125 ml sunflower oil
> 200 g caster sugar
> 2 large eggs
> 1 tsp vanilla extract
> 3 mashed ripe bananas
> 175 g plain flour
> 1 tsp bicarbonate of soda
> ½ tsp ground cinnamon

Turn the mixture into a lined loaf tin (e.g. 900 g/2 lb tin) and bake at 180°C (160°C fan)/350°F/gas mark 4 for about one hour. Take it out and let it cool.

Final, Primal Recipes

Making banana bread is incredibly simple, and simplicity is a central feature of cooking and eating primally. After all, cavemen wouldn't have had access to a million different superfoods or specialist oils from around the world; they could only use what was in their immediate surroundings. For those of us who have less than advanced kitchen skills, it's off-putting to read lengthy lists of ingredients, and complicated preparation and cooking techniques.

Even if you're not an adventurous cook, you can still make delicious meals. I've learnt that keeping it simple is both satisfying and primal. It also cuts down on waste. Here are a few tasty, primal ideas for meat-eaters, soup lovers, pasta fiends and veggies alike.

Steak and blue cheese sandwiches (serves 2)

1 large ciabatta loaf
2 rib-eye steaks (around 200 g each)
115 g Gorgonzola cheese, sliced
Olive oil, salt and black pepper

Bake or warm the ciabatta, then remove from oven and leave to cool. Cut the loaf in half and split each half horizontally. Heat griddle pan (or grill) until hot. Brush the steaks with olive oil and lay them on the griddle pan. Cook for 2–3 minutes on each side, depending on the thickness of the steaks. Cook for longer if you prefer them well done. Remove the steaks and set aside for a few minutes. Place them in the sandwiches with the blue cheese, and season with salt and black pepper.

Tuscan bean soup

2 x 400 g tins of chopped tomatoes (ideally with mixed herbs)
250 g cavolo nero leaves or savoy cabbage
1 tin of cannellini beans (400 g)
Extra-virgin olive oil, salt and black pepper

Tip the chopped tomatoes into a large pan and add one tin of cold water. Season with salt and pepper, and bring to the boil, then simmer. Shred the cavolo nero/cabbage leaves and add them to the pan. Partially cover the pan and simmer gently for around 15 minutes, until the cabbage is tender. Drain and rinse the cannellini beans, add to the pan and warm through for another few minutes. Add more seasoning to taste and then serve in warm bowls. Drizzle each one with olive oil, serving with ciabatta bread. This traditional Tuscan peasant soup is primal and hugely satisfying!

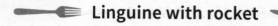

Linguine with rocket

350 g fresh or dried linguine
A large bunch of rocket (150 g) shredded or torn,
with stalks removed
75 g Parmesan cheese, freshly grated
Extra-virgin olive oil, salt and black pepper

Cook the linguine in boiling water until al dente, then drain. Heat the olive oil in the pasta pan, and add the drained linguine, followed by the rocket. Toss over a medium heat for one or two minutes, until the rocket is wilted. Tip the pasta into a warm bowl, add half the Parmesan and another drizzle of olive oil, salt and black pepper to taste. Toss and serve with the remaining Parmesan.

There are so many simple pasta dishes like this: penne, crushed tomatoes and basil; spaghetti with broccoli; chilli spaghetti, or with butter, garlic and cheese – just as they serve it in Italy.

Grilled aubergine, mint and couscous salad

1 large aubergine
115 g couscous
Garlic, chopped fresh mint, olive oil,
salt and black pepper

Preheat the grill. Cut the aubergine into chunky strips and sprinkle them with olive oil, salt and black pepper. Spread the aubergine strips on a baking sheet, and grill them for 5–6 minutes, turning occasionally until golden brown. Prepare the couscous with garlic and chopped mint. Stir the grilled aubergine strips into the couscous, add more oil if needed, and garnish with mint leaves. Toss thoroughly and enjoy!

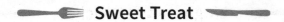

Sweet Treat

Lastly, for the sweet tooth which lurks within us all, here is a simple recipe for Honey Biscuits (makes 30).

> 120 g butter
> 120 g caster sugar
> 1 ½ tbsp honey
> 1 egg yolk
> 1 tsp cinnamon
> 180 g self-raising flour
> A little extra cinnamon and caster sugar
> for dusting on top of biscuits.

Heat the oven to 180°C/350°F/gas mark 4.

Mix the butter and sugar together in a bowl until well-blended and creamy, then add in the honey and the egg yolk, until thoroughly blended. Add the cinnamon and the flour, then mix into a soft dough. If it's too sticky to handle, add a small amount of flour.

Shape 1 tsp of dough into a ball, roll it in the (extra) sugar and cinnamon, and place on a greased baking tray. Continue shaping little dough balls until all the mixture is used up.

Leave a space between each dough ball, because the biscuits will spread in the oven.

Bake for 12–15 minutes, until golden brown.

Take the biscuits out of the oven and leave to settle on the tray for a few minutes. Then transfer to cake rack or plate to cool.

The benefits of eating clean, unprocessed ingredients that have come straight from the earth are obvious: better digestion and energy levels, clearer skin, and improved mood, concentration and sleep – and yes, a stable, healthy weight. Eating primally is not a magic bullet for weight loss, but it's primal in the best way: good for you and good for the planet.

Adopting a primal attitude quickly becomes a virtuous cycle, whereby you learn to love the foods that do you good. Cutting back on salt, sugar and artificial ingredients will wake up your taste buds, and re-accustom them to the more delicate delights of herbs and spices. Eating primally puts you back in touch with freshness and flavour, with your body's natural appetite, and with the seasonal cycles of the Earth. Whether you're thinking of your own health or the planet, or a combination of the two, primal eating will boost, heal and nourish you from the inside out.

Chapter 7
Primal Hunger

How often have you heard the advice: 'Eat when you're hungry, stop when you're full'?

It's simple, logical and we all know it works. And yet sometimes the simplest advice is the hardest to follow.

Hungry for What?

If every time you feel lonely, you bury the feeling by binge-eating – what happens? If you deal with your sense of abandonment by depriving yourself of food – what happens? One thing's for sure: it doesn't sort out the root cause. When we suppress painful emotions, or transfer them into a disordered relationship with food, we end up in a mess.

Too often we confuse physical needs and emotional feelings, sublimating them into eating. Getting back in touch with your primal hungers is the only way to get them straightened out.

There *are* occasions when physical actions can relieve difficult emotions. I find that a session of kick-boxing, for example, calms me when I'm het up; a swim clears my head when I'm feeling upset. But at some point we need to deal with the emotion itself: it won't go away otherwise, no matter how hard we try to punch/swim/starve it out of us. And food may be wonderful, but it's never going to solve a fear of intimacy, an inferiority complex or a childhood trauma.

People channel their emotions into other problem behaviours too: gambling, shopping or self-harming, and sometimes in drug or alcohol addiction. But food is overwhelmingly the commonest: it's widely available, socially acceptable, and it tastes good. Until overeating or under-eating goes too far, and becomes a form of self-sabotage.

Our behaviour around food is often subconscious; often it goes back many years. Whether it's overeating or under-eating, we don't consciously choose this way of dealing with problems. And of course, it's not logical: people don't overeat because they're greedy or want to be overweight. At the other end of the spectrum, people with anorexia nervosa don't starve themselves because they're not hungry or necessarily want to be underweight. The roots of disordered eating go far deeper than that. As the US author Geneen Roth puts it, 'People often feel that who they are is not enough, and eat to try to make that feeling go away.' Somewhere along the way, when we're repeatedly using food to suppress our feelings or to punish ourselves, we lose the ability to tune into our bodies.

It's not surprising that many of us have lost touch with our primal 'hungry' and 'full' instincts. Behaviours such as dieting and overeating repeatedly override our internal hunger cues, and we struggle to tune in to them. We get confused about what and when to eat, and how much.

When you tune in to, rather than override, your natural hunger cues, you'll find they're the safest guide to eating the right amount.

Eat Like a Child

As a child, it's likely that you intuitively ate when you were hungry, and stopped when you were full. You may think you never had this ability, but you probably did. Before food became a battleground of greed and guilt, bingeing and fasting, excess and shame, punishment and reward. Before you got bombarded with sociocultural mixed messages and advertisements. Before you associated food with weight or the size or shape or desirability of your body. You ate the right amount to satisfy your primal hunger.

As adults, many of us lose this intuitive relationship with food. I had anorexia for ten years, so I know what a struggle it can be. For me, admitting that I needed food felt like an admission of failure. 'Giving in' to hunger seemed weak. What I aspired to, throughout the long process of recovery, was to learn to trust my body's primal appetites and regain that natural, childlike attitude to food: hunger and appetite and pleasure.

Looking back, I can see that physical hunger wasn't the problem at all. I was no more or less greedy (or deserving) than anyone else.

A whole load of other emotions had got in the way, and they felt overwhelming, and the only way I could keep control of the whole thing blowing up in my face (or so I thought) was to control what I ate.

Finding our way back to a more primal relationship with our hungers, both physical and emotional, can be immensely rewarding. These primal needs, appetites and emotions lie at the heart of what make us human. Our bodies are constantly sending us signals: not only about danger (e.g. *don't step into the traffic*) but feelings too: *when he said that, I felt hurt.*

If you struggle with over- or under-eating, you'll be aware that it's not solving anything. The most powerful tool in your fight for a happy, healthy relationship with food is understanding and accepting your different hungers. Once you learn to recognise and respond to what your body needs, physically and emotionally, everything else falls into place. Let's take a look at some of the different hungers we all experience.

Stomach Hunger

Stomach hunger involves an interaction between the digestive system, endocrine system and brain. You experience a hollowness or emptiness in the stomach, an ache or rumbling inside. You may feel tired and it may be hard to concentrate. This is genuine physical hunger, and when you start to refuel with food, your body will respond by feeling better.

If you don't respond to hunger with food, the physical symptoms intensify. You may get bad stomach pains and start to feel irritable or short-tempered. Your blood sugar is low, and this may cause headaches or dizziness. You may feel shaky and weak.

At this point, you're really ravenous and feel like you could eat anything. It's not a good idea to get this hungry, because you're less likely to make balanced nutritional choices. Unhealthy fast food begins to look irresistible; a take-away pizza or family-sized bar of chocolate are more readily available and will fill the gap more quickly than cooking a meal with fresh ingredients.

The point about stomach hunger is to respond to it when it's manageable. Far better to eat a sensible amount when your hunger is keen than to wait until you're starving, when you may be at risk of bingeing. Basically, you should be looking forward to your next meal, but not so ravenous that you're ready to commit an act of cannibalism. I'm sure you're familiar with the term 'hangry'!

Knowing When to Stop

In order to avoid getting out-of-control hungry, it's important to pay attention to your body. When you're feeling relaxed and eating calmly (i.e. not desperately cramming it in), you'll notice clear primal signals from your brain and stomach as soon as you've eaten enough. Here's how it works:

- hunger and fullness are regulated by the hypothalamus
- when you've eaten enough, signals are sent to the hypothalamus to indicate fullness
- your stomach feels comfortable: not empty but not over-stuffed
- your body feels 'satiated' or satisfied.

However, it takes around 20 minutes for the stomach to signal to the brain that it's satiated. Often, we eat beyond the point of fullness because we're not paying attention to our bodies. It's a good idea to slow down when eating, chew each mouthful and listen to when your body is satisfied. Pay attention: even before the fullness signals, when you've had the right amount of food, you'll notice that you feel calmer and more energised. Don't rush yourself: allow your food to go down. Sit at the table and see how you feel. Remember that your body will tell you if you've had enough or you need a little more. Tune in, trusting that primal feeling.

Signs of Overeating

- You're eating so quickly that you're barely chewing or tasting the food.
- You're swallowing mechanically, but you're not enjoying the food anymore.

You're starting to feel physically uncomfortable: this may be a sensation of pressure or fullness in your stomach, even nausea.

You feel lethargic or sluggish after eating: the thrill of consuming all that food is quickly replaced by guilt.

As well as physical discomfort, how does your head feel? When you've eaten the right amount of good food, you'll feel content and nourished. When you've overeaten, you may experience shame or regret: you've consumed without enjoying it, and now you wish you hadn't.

Remember as a child being told not to bolt your food? Turns out there's a good physiological reason why...

Researcher Dr Alexander Kokkinos (Laiko General Hospital in Athens) divided participants into two groups: the first had five minutes to eat 300 ml of ice cream and the second had 30 minutes. He found that the slow eaters had higher concentrations of two hormones – called PYY and GLP-1 – than the fast eaters. PYY and GLP-1 hormones are released by the stomach after a meal to tell the brain that it is full. This could indicate that people who eat more quickly aren't warned by these hormones that it is time to stop and, consequently, eat too much.

Fast eaters also feel hungry again sooner because it takes the brain up to 20 minutes to process the fact that it has consumed food, and for the stomach to signal to the brain that it's satiated. Bolting our food strips us of our ability to remember the sensation of eating. (*Journal of Clinical Endocrinology & Metabolism*, 2010).

In order to regain our primal hunger, we need to understand what else might be getting in the way, such as a range of routines, habits and emotions which can vary widely between individuals. Do you recognise any of these reasons for overeating?

- You've been brought up not to leave anything on your plate.

- You're clearing leftovers from children's meals.

- You don't want to waste the food.

- You're bored.

- You've stuck to the new diet all day and now you could eat a horse.

- You don't want to offend the person who cooked it.

- It's a buffet situation (complicated!).

- It's the weekend; you deserve a treat.

- You're watching TV and fancy a snack.

- You're at the cinema, which means popcorn.

- You're eating out for work.

- You can't sleep.

- You're exhausted and need some energy.

- It's a birthday and it would be rude not to.

- The food looks and smells tempting.

- It's just there…

… And a million other reasons! They're all valid, and totally understandable, but they're not really stomach hunger.

No Blame, No Shame

Emotional eating – especially bingeing – is fraught with feelings of shame, blame and even self-disgust. Time to forgive yourself. Overeating is not unusual, and being a bit indulgent doesn't make you a greedy person. Neither does it make you bad or worthless. Humans habitually overeat; we live in a world of abundance and it can be hard to find the control switch.

False Hungers

Instead of feeling guilty or ashamed, take back control by learning to identify those false hungers instead.

Mouth hunger: you're tempted by delicious-looking or delicious-smelling food. Smell is an incredibly potent sense: up to 80 per cent of what we taste actually comes from smell. Good aromas trigger your taste buds and your mouth starts to water, regardless of whether you're actually hungry. Supermarkets are clever at playing on this – what could be more tempting than the smell of freshly baked bread? This is why it's unwise to go shopping when you're ravenous.

Eye (or visual) hunger: again, this is when you're visually drawn to delicious food and convinced that you need to eat even though you're not actually hungry. Have you ever found yourself gazing in the window of a French patisserie, taste buds watering? Or salivating during cookery programmes or while reading recipe books?

Clock hunger: 1 p.m. = lunch and 7.30 p.m. = dinner time, right? Perhaps you're not particularly hungry but you're eating because 'it's time'. Often we eat with others, automatically, without even registering whether we're hungry at that moment. This is common at work or school, where there are set times for lunch or breaks, so we have to eat then, rather than when we really want to. Try experimenting with your food clock, waiting until you're properly hungry to eat.

Thirst: dehydration slows down our energy levels, making us feel below par. It can also make us feel hungry – when we're actually thirsty. When the body is dehydrated, it needs fluids rather than food. Increase your intake of water and herbal teas. Fruit and vegetables are another great source of healthy fluids.

Fatigue: insufficient sleep plays havoc with our moods and our appetite. When energy levels are low, it's tempting to reach for something to boost your blood sugar, often a short-term fix. However, caffeinated drinks and sugary snacks aren't the long-term solution.

The nutritionist Petronella Ravenshear explains how sleep quality can directly affect our hunger: 'Poor sleep adversely affects the appetite hormones leptin and ghrelin. After a restless night leptin, which makes us feel full, goes down, and ghrelin, which stimulates our appetite, goes up. On a regular basis that leads to overeating.'

When your body is tired, it needs rest, not food. If sleep isn't an option, healthy snacks like fresh fruit, carrots and hummus or nuts and seeds will keep you going longer than junk food.

Heart hunger: emotions affect people in different ways: some lose their appetites completely, while others try to fill the void with food. If you're feeling lonely or upset, the ache or emptiness inside can be easily confused with physical hunger. However, bingeing or starving won't really solve it. Try to avoid eating when you're in a highly emotional state: far better to talk problems through, and then eat.

Mindless Eating

Studies show that eating while distracted can result in a 40 per cent greater calorie intake than usual. Modern life is full of distractions, most commonly digital ones – fiddling with smartphones, working, watching TV, and so on – all coming between us and our body's internal cues.

It's hardly surprising that this kind of mindless eating leads to excess calories and weight gain. You're so busy doing something else, such as rushing down the street, taking calls and replying to emails, that the food fails to register. You don't feel like you've eaten properly – because you haven't stopped for a meal – and often overeat as a result. During research, crisp-eaters consumed more if they ate crisps out of a bag or a tube than if they poured a finite amount into a bowl. Their brain didn't tell them to stop. Similarly, researchers at the University of Surrey found that participants who ate while they walked consumed more throughout the day than those snacking while stationary.

Focusing on your food, also known as mindful eating (or not-eating-while-totally-distracted-by-your-phone), is really worth the effort. Making time to eat, and concentrating on your plate, also leads to greater enjoyment of your food and a healthy sense of satiation. If you don't feel satiated, after all, you're more likely to keep going with the crisps, biscuits, cakes, long after you're full. You also absorb and digest your food better when you have time to chew, pause and breathe between mouthfuls.

13 golden rules of primal, mindful eating.

1. Don't eat while standing up or walking along the street.

2. Avoid eating while working, chatting on the phone or being otherwise distracted.

3. Share and talk. If you're at work, sit down with colleagues; if you're at home, sit with your partner or family. Meals are about conversation and sharing, as well as refuelling.

4. Use plates and cutlery, tables and chairs. Use plates of a reasonable size and don't pile them too high. Don't eat straight out of takeaway containers – serve yourself a reasonable portion on a plate.

5. If you have time, light candles and use napkins. It's all about making meals a pleasurable occasion.

6. Eat (and talk) – don't tweet. No one on social media needs to know what you're eating.

7. Switch off the television and other gadgets. When you're transfixed by a screen, your attention is not on your food, and you risk overeating.

8. Break the habit of snacking while watching, whether that's TV or at the cinema. You don't need food to enjoy a box-set!

9. The same goes for those moreish tubes of crisps: remember that 'once you pop you can't stop'. It may feel strange to put crisps in a bowl, or put chunks of chocolate on a plate, but it will stop you polishing off the lot.

10. Don't bolt your food: it takes around 20 minutes for your brain to register that you're full. Remember: it's a meal, not a race. Research shows that slow eaters consume 2 oz of food per minute, while fast eaters eat 3.1 oz. You save up to 70 calories by slowing down.

11. Try not to pick at food while you're cooking. Don't hoover up leftovers while clearing away your kids' dinner either. No need to waste good food: instead, keep it for another meal, use it as

the basis for next day's office lunchbox or chuck any scrappy bits on a compost heap.

12. Chew each bite properly: remember that good digestion begins in your mouth. Appreciate the look, smell and taste of your food: consciously savour the colours and aromas.

13. Make time after meals for a cup of mint or green tea, or your preferred *digestif*. This will signal to your body that you've finished eating and are pleasantly satiated, and it aids digestion.

Expert Perspective

Lesley Jefferson, clinical hypnotherapist, uses mindfulness to help clients who are struggling with emotional eating. She finds that the benefits go far beyond weight management, spreading into her clients' lives more widely. She explains:

Mindful eating is beneficial to those who are tired of the yo-yo cycle of weight loss and gain – and those who are ready to take responsibility for getting back to a healthy weight. Once they accept that diets don't work and there's no perfect body pill, they're on the right road. And once they start to feel in control again and, to their joyful surprise, start to enjoy their food again, they realise they have found something that lasts a lifetime.

Mindful eating is often tougher for people who are used to consuming a lot of processed foods. The blissful combinations of salt, fat and sugar – that aren't found anywhere in nature – give the brain's reward centre a big buzz. That makes us want to prolong the pleasure – it's not hard to eat these foods beyond satiety.

Mindful eating is a skill that takes time, practice and attention. It's possible to get a long way just by eating real food, and regularly asking the question 'am I hungry'?

There are many simple strategies to avoid the raging hunger which tends to lead to unhealthy eating, and to reconnect with your natural, healthy appetite.

Breaking Your Fast

What could be more primal than the first meal of the day? After a night of resting and repairing, you need to recharge those cells to get ready for the day ahead. Just as you refuel your car with petrol, you need to replenish your body with high-quality nutrition. The 'blue light' of the morning hours also kick-starts the body's metabolism, thus explaining why morning hunger can feel intensely primal: literally, a breaking of the fast.

Breakfast is also essential for maintaining a healthy body weight. Studies show that those who regularly eat breakfast are more successful at both losing weight and keeping it off. As Milton Stokes, the Chief Dietitian for St. Barnabas Hospital in New York explains: 'People skip breakfast thinking they're cutting calories, but by mid-morning and lunch that person is starved. Breakfast skippers replace calories during the day with mindless nibbling and bingeing at lunch and dinner. They set themselves up for failure.'

Whether it's hot or cold, porridge and berries, fruit salad, yogurt and cereal, or eggs or fish on wholegrain toast, a healthy breakfast will replenish your energy reserves and kick-start your metabolism. Embrace your primal hunger, and 'breakfast like a king'. It really is the most important meal of the day.

Primal Portions

Portion size is one of the simplest ways to tackle overeating. The average size of dinner plates has grown in recent times, and dimensions still differ across the world. The average UK dinner plate today measures around 11–12 inches across, whereas a few decades ago plates measured 7–9 inches. In Europe, the average plate measures 9 inches, while some American restaurants use plates that are around 13 inches in diameter.

Which are you: European- or American-sized? Do your dinner plates resemble frisbees, or even dustbin lids? Most of us are hardwired to fill our plates (sometimes piling them high) and to finish everything on them. Using something a little smaller could help to cut down on those rugby-player size portions of pasta!

When you're looking at portion sizes, bear in mind that different foods should be consumed in different amounts. Divide your plate into roughly one-quarter of complex carbs, one-quarter of quality protein and a half of vegetables.

Dieting Let-down

> 66 *Probably nothing in the world arouses more false hopes than the first four hours of a diet.* 99

This comment from the Irish dramatist Samuel Beckett is funny, painful and deeply relatable. Diets promise a new start – a whole new you – but usually fail to deliver. Eating too much, too little or the wrong stuff goes a whole lot deeper than a shiny new app, book or celebrity endorsement.

Added to our personal emotional maelstroms are the daily, relentless, conflicting messages that we receive: the newest miracle diet, the latest food fad, what weight and shape our bodies *should* be. Every week brings different advice: eat mostly meat, use butter and cream, drink juice three days a week or avoid gluten like the plague – it's confusing, inconsistent and exhausting. If you're fed up with yo-yo dieting, it's time to reject the mentality of deprivation and restriction.

Restrictive diets really don't work. Up to 95 per cent of dieters regain the lost weight and more. Start again with a wholesome, inclusive attitude to food. When nothing is forbidden, you can enjoy a little of everything. Balance may sound boring, but it's essential.

Eat Green, Eat Clean

I promised there would be no talk of diets or weight loss in this book. But here are some simple, primal guidelines which are good for you and good for the planet. You don't have to follow all the principles all the time, but they may form a positive basis for a greener, cleaner eating regime.

- Choose food as close to its natural state as possible. The guiding principle should be the quality and freshness of your produce – not points or calories.

- This means eating more fresh fruit and vegetables, nuts and seeds, and organic meat and fish.

- It also means avoiding processed, low-fat, fat-free or refined foods.

- Don't deprive yourself. Anyone who has ever been on a strict diet knows the risks of restriction and bingeing: banning certain 'bad' foods or whole groups and then craving them like mad.

- By permitting yourself to eat anything, within reason, you avoid the cycle of miserable hunger and guilty splurge.

- Don't ignore cravings. If you're longing for some chocolate, choose a raw or organic dark type, containing 70 per cent cocoa solids or higher. As well as giving you that chocolate hit, it's a great source of antioxidants.

- Practise moderation and pursue variety. Eating a wide and diverse diet will give you more vitamins, minerals, phytonutrients and amino acids. Everything can be enjoyed in moderation, as long as it's natural and unprocessed.

- Remember that nothing is intrinsically evil, and no food should be 'banned' from your diet.

- But do glance at labels: do you recognise the ingredients? Try to limit your intake of artificial additives and preservatives. They raise your blood sugar levels, and then leave you craving more.

- Experiment with herbs and spices for flavouring – usually far tastier than anything heavily processed.

The beauty of eating primally is that nothing needs to be forbidden. You can basically make healthy versions of almost anything: chips and burgers, stir-fries, raw dips and even chocolate brownies. Remember: you don't need to count calories or deny yourself treats – just keep them natural. When you're eating nutritionally rich foods, your body feels satisfied and well-nourished.

Whatever you eat, replace: 'How many calories does it contain?' with 'How much healthy nutrition will I get from this?'

Diet Backlash

There's no doubt that we've been controlled by the diet, calorie-counting, weight-loss industry for decades now. However, the good news is that, finally, there are signs we may be reaching peak diet-hysteria. Increasingly, we're rejecting the body-weight fascism, regaining our sanity and going back to basics. Respected nutritionists and scientists (those without miracle diets or supplements to sell) are speaking up for normal eating again. Yes, that means gluten, dairy, fat and even some sugar, but everything in moderation: lots of fresh fruit and vegetables, meat and fish if you choose it, carbs and protein, plus sensible treats.

> **Vicky, 36:** I'm so tired of reading articles and books from 'health experts' telling me what I should or shouldn't be eating. After 18 years of trying every diet possible, several eating disorders, and rock-bottom self-esteem, I'm ashamed to say I let myself become consumed by these fads instead of concentrating on more important things. We live in a world where people are starving, yet we're agonising over a kale smoothie or a burger for lunch...

Faddy diets are just that: FADS. Here's why a primal, balanced attitude to eating makes sense.

- Cutting out whole food groups throws your body out of balance.

- Demonising specific foods is also nonsensical, and makes you crave them even more.

- Fat-free products are often high in refined sugar, and deprive your body of essential fats.

- Carb-free diets are often high in saturated fats and/or excessive protein.

- Juicing, fasting or starving is unsustainable, unhealthy and not particularly effective for weight loss.

- Nutritional variety, regular exercise and sensible portion control are way more effective than dieting.

- Deprivation doesn't work. The healthiest people tend to love their food!

Understand Your Primal Hunger

When you understand your body's different kinds of hunger, you can respect rather than fear them. Here are some simple ways to stop messing with your primal hunger.

Cut back on snacks: we're surrounded by 'eating opportunities' – look at the average high street or airport – but our primal ancestors were not forever snacking. We don't need to be topping up on calories all the time. Learning to recognise your hunger is important! Diets or fasts can mess with the simple signals of satiety and hunger. Avoid constant grazing on smoothies or cereal bars. Leave decent gaps between eating, so that you feel moderately hungry when you come to your next good, nutritious meal.

Slow down: when you're eating, slow down. Take time to savour the food in front of you. What can you taste? How do the flavours interact? Focus on the different textures of crunch and smooth. When you're rushed – or feeling guilt or shame – you cram food in, barely tasting it. It's better for your digestion (and your heart) to enjoy every mouthful. Mindful eating recommends chewing each mouthful up to 60 times (a bit extreme!) but you can see the point. If you swallow food without tasting it, you won't feel nourished or satiated.

Focus on food: when you're not snacking you can focus on three really satisfying and nutritious meals per day. Set aside time for them: don't eat when you're rushed or distracted. Ideally, you should stop and do nothing but eat (and breathe). You can talk too, as long as it's to actual eating companions who are with you. Avoid eating while driving, working, watching TV or talking on the phone. When people become present during meals, they tend to eat less overall, and enjoy their food more.

Green-light Foods for Primal Energy

Eating for health, strength and power is liberating: deciding to eat well is joyous and brave. Food is life, energy and fuel for our tanks, and if we want to be strong, we need to keep those tanks topped up with quality fuel. Having struggled with anorexia for a long time, I understand how important it is to feel that what you're eating is good, natural, wholesome and nourishing. Silly as it sounds, it helps to be reassured that eating plentiful amounts of real food won't make you gain weight – because it really won't.

Here are some of the nutritious foods I include regularly: almonds, walnuts, cashew and Brazil nuts, sunflower and pumpkin seeds, whole grains, brown rice, quinoa, legumes, chickpeas, flaxseed, coconut or olive oil, broccoli, cherry tomatoes, asparagus, bananas, apples, blueberries, cherries and Greek yogurt.

These are wholesome, slow-release, energy-boosting foods, overflowing with nutritional goodness. They will increase your energy levels, and give you clear skin, shiny hair and a spring in your step... Proceed without guilt.

Final Word: When to Get Help

Emotional eating is quite common – after all, food is inextricably linked with our deepest experiences of nurture, family, celebration, reward, comfort and safety. From the moment we're born, food is the reassurance that we're being loved and cared for. To some extent, everyone's an emotional eater! However, if the problems go deeper than this, do seek professional advice.

It's important to recognise that you're not alone: eating just the right amount is a struggle for many people. Needing help has nothing to do with your actual weight – you are not undeserving if you're overeating and you don't need to be underweight to merit professional help. Emotions and narratives around food can be buried very deep, and it can be helpful to work through these with an expert. A specially trained therapist will be able to help with you a range of emotional eating issues, from anorexia to bulimia to binge-eating disorders and everything in between.

Don't be afraid of your primal, physical hunger. We're fortunate in the West that there's plenty of food to go around. However, when we're constantly snacking or dieting, our blood sugar levels tend to spike and plummet confusingly. Once you start eating three nutritious meals a day, you give your stomach enough to digest – and a chance to rest between meals. Remember the mantra: eat when you're hungry; stop when you're full.

You should also seek medical advice for physical concerns: if you habitually feel full after only a few mouthfuls or you're constantly hungry no matter how much you consume. There can be a range of reasons: stress, illness, depression and some medications can all increase or decrease your appetite.

Finally, don't forget that as human beings, our metabolisms, activity levels, eating behaviours and tastes are individual – we all require different types and quantities of food. Stop worrying about diets, mirrors, bathroom scales or what others are consuming. Primal eating gives you the confidence to welcome, rather than fear, your natural appetite. A human who is not hungry may be sick, listless, even dying. Getting hungry is the most primal sign that your body is healthy and active, and wants energy.

Hunger is an opportunity to explore the world of flavours out there, and refuel your body in the most pleasurable way. There is no need to replace real food with food-like substances: safe ingredients will never do you harm. Milkshakes, pills or powders are no substitute for the primal pleasure of foraging and shopping, cooking, experimenting and eating, whether alone or with others. Tune into your primal hunger, listen to your body and eat well for you.

Chapter 8
Primal and Meat-free

❝ One day our meat-eating habits are going to be looked at in the same way as we look at our smoking habits in the 1970s. There will be die-hards that do it but no one will be ignoring the fact that it is lowering our life expectancy. ❞

Dan Buettner is a US explorer who claims to have found the secret of life – or at least the food eaten by those who live the longest. After a decade studying the lifestyle and diets of the longest-lived communities around the world, he wrote a book called *The Blue Zones Solution: Eating and Living Like the World's Healthiest People.*

What was special about the diets in these so-called Blue Zones? In a word: beans. Buettner argues that beans are 'the world's greatest longevity foods'. His research found that these long-lifers are eating on average a cup of beans a day, of any and every variety: fava, soy, black beans and lentils are fundamental to healthy living and the cornerstone of every longevity diet. Beans are high in fibre, vitamins and micronutrients, and an excellent replacement for animal protein. They also create far healthier gut bacteria than meat, helping to lower inflammation (linked to ageing) and prevent obesity.

Another notable feature of these populations is that they eat very little meat: on average around once a week. Around 95 per cent of their diet comes from plants or plant products: meat is seen as a rare treat rather than a staple ingredient.

These long-lived populations, found in areas as diverse as Greece, Japan, California, Sardinia and Costa Rica, have significantly lower rates of heart disease, diabetes and dementia. Interestingly, their diets aren't intentionally vegan or veggie, or healthy – it's the way they naturally eat, and their longevity is a natural result.

Even better, these people aren't impossibly saintly: they enjoy moderate amounts of red wine and drink strong coffee. Neither are they exercise freaks; instead, they stay fit with natural movement in their everyday lives, such as housework and walking to work.

Superfoods eaten regularly in these regions include vegetables, fruits, beans, grains, nuts/seeds, lean protein, dairy, oils, coffee, tea, red wine and water – plus seasonings such as garlic, herbs, turmeric and honey.

In recent years the term 'primal' has been appropriated by the Paleo community to describe a diet based primarily around meat and fish, the so-called 'caveman' diet. It therefore follows that a vegetarian or vegan can't eat primally, right? Being 'primal' and meat-free is an oxymoron, right?

Wrong. If eating primally – with the emphasis on natural, unprocessed foods – appeals to you, as it does to me, you can absolutely do this without eating meat. If you're looking to cut down on your meat consumption, or give it up altogether, you can do that too. The Earth is abundant with crops, fruit and vegetables which will supply all your nutritional needs, without an abattoir, butchers' block or fishing trawler in sight.

A Word About Paleo

The Paleo model is based on the concept of foraging and hunter-gathering, with the emphasis on meat, fish, game, berries and nuts. It includes fats found in avocados, nuts and seeds, olive oil, fish oil and coconut oil. The regime minimises grains and carbohydrates, sugar, wheat, transfats and industrialised omega-6 fats, and contains little or no dairy. Paleos believe that the human digestive system is not designed to cope with highly processed, high-calorie foods, and that insoluble grain fibre causes obesity, heart disease, diabetes, inflammation, irritable bowel syndrome and countless other modern afflictions.

The Paleo movement has resulted in specialist cafés and restaurants opening across Europe and the US. However, the evidence is sketchy. Archaeologists cannot say with certainty what our primal ancestors ate, and they don't all believe that grains were completely absent from early man's diet. While fossilised bones, teeth and cooking implements have survived, archaeological traces of the actual food have not. Even though researchers know enough to make some generalisations about human diets in the Palaeolithic period, the details are not precise. Exactly what proportions of meat and vegetables did different species eat? It's not clear. Just how far back were our ancestors eating grains and dairy? Perhaps far earlier than we initially thought. What's certain is that in the Palaeolithic era, the human diet varied immensely by geography, season and opportunity.

This is not to dismiss the Paleo approach altogether. There may not be solid scientific evidence, but the philosophy makes some sense. In the West we consume carbs and grains at almost every meal – toast, sandwiches, pasta, potatoes, rice, biscuits – and digestive complaints such as IBS and bloating are common. Clearly, our guts are not designed to cope with excessive amount of insoluble grain fibre. Paleo eating aims to replace all these refined ingredients with natural food, and that can only be a good thing.

Primal Appetites

People have all sorts of reasons for giving up, or cutting down, on meat. These range from health concerns to individual tastes to ethical considerations and concern for animal welfare. Whatever the reason, there is no doubt that the growing consumption of meat among an ever-expanding global population is taking its toll on the environment.

The facts about worldwide meat consumption are startling: the UK eats over 80 kg of meat per person per year, around double the global average. To put that in context, Americans consume an average of 125 kg of meat per person and Indians an average of 5 kg per person. And yet most omnivores claim that they 'eat hardly any meat' – conveniently forgetting the bacon sandwich they devoured for breakfast, the ham sandwich at lunch and the chicken curry for dinner.

The Truth About Meat

In 2013 the horse meat scandal erupted with the discovery that unidentified animal matter was being widely passed off as beef across the UK and Europe. Equine DNA was discovered in frozen beef burgers, sausages and lasagne, as well as high levels of pig DNA and other undeclared meat substances. This fuelled the move towards eating less meat, or at least an increase in public demand for greater transparency and traceability in the food supply chain.

The reality of modern factory farming is shocking. Most of us suspect that conditions are pretty awful; maybe we've seen a documentary about abattoirs or battery chickens, or heard about the mass transportation of live animals. Even those who don't eat meat shy away from knowing too much – perhaps because we feel powerless to change things? The real, unvarnished truth can be distressing (try reading Jonathan Safran Foer's *Eating Animals*).

Taking a primal attitude to the world around you, including other species, means caring about how others are treated. None of this cruelty is necessary: animals were not kept in such conditions in the past. Whether or not you eat meat, their lives – and deaths – should at least be humane. Sadly, this is not the case. Take the culling of newborn chicks. As male chicks have no egg-laying value and are not suitable for meat production, they need to be destroyed once hatched. Culling methods include cervical dislocation (breaking the neck), asphyxiation by carbon dioxide, electrocution (a new method which is considered cheap, reliable and humane) or even suffocation in plastic bags. One of the most popular current techniques is maceration, where live chicks are thrown into a high-speed grinder.

It's not just male chicks. Animals suffer close confinement, semi-conscious transportation across long distances, routine use of antibiotics, hormones and drugs to artificially accelerate growth, and mutilation such as breaking of beaks and docking of tails. By any measure, this is an inhumane regime of pain, hunger, disease, fear and distress. The mistreatment of animals is widespread – not in a few rogue farms, but in the mainstream farming industry. It gets to the point where the only way you can eat factory-farmed meat is not to think about it – or not to care.

Terms such as *free range, farm-fresh, grass-fed, pasture-raised* or *welfare-friendly* have become virtually meaningless. Anyone can use these terms. *Free range*, for example, doesn't actually mean free to roam around: under EU guidelines, chickens that spend their lives confined inside massive industrial barns can be labelled as *free range*, as long as there is 'access to' a small outside area.

But what if you're ethical and caring, and want to eat produce which has been reared in a humane way? Who can we trust?

I'm not here to lecture you – what we eat is a personal choice. But shouldn't we all become more involved in the process of our food production, asking hard questions and boycotting inhumane practices? We may *feel* powerless – because this stuff just arrives on our supermarket shelves, with misleading labels and false assurances of welfare standards – but we have immense power.

Couldn't we demand a more primal approach to animal rearing and slaughter? Of course, 'nature is red in tooth and claw', and our Palaeolithic ancestors were no panda-cuddling vegans. They chased, killed and gobbled up those wild oxen, deer and cave bears. But at least it was a level playing field: the animals lived free and died naturally in the cycle of predator and prey. They were not pumped full of unnecessary antibiotics, crammed in tiny cages or chucked into industrial mincers at birth. They were not force-fed until they were so obese that their legs collapsed under their own weight.

On top of the ethical and health issues, and welfare concerns about intensive factory farming, our meat addiction exerts a huge toll on the environment. Around a third of the world's cereal harvest – enough to feed three billion people – is fed to farm animals. Then there's the pollution from methane: worldwide livestock farming generates around 18 per cent of the planet's greenhouse gas emissions. (By comparison, all the world's cars, trains, planes and boats account for a combined 13 per cent of greenhouse gas emissions.) Annually, a single cow emits around 120 kg of methane (in belching and flatulence) compared with a human being's annual 0.12 kg. And, molecule for molecule, methane has a much greater warming effect than carbon dioxide.

The Cost of Meat Production

Global meat production is projected to more than double from 229 million tonnes in the year 2000 to 465 million tonnes by 2050. The sheer amount of grain and water needed to produce all this livestock is staggering. Here are the estimated costs of grain needed to make 1 kilo of meat:

around 7 kilos of grain to make 1 kilo of beef
around 4 kilos of grain to make 1 kilo of pork
around 2 kilos of grain to make 1 kilo of chicken.

Then there's the vast water footprint of meat production: in the current global water crisis, this matters. The production of vegetables, nuts and grains consumes far less water than animal products. If you want to reduce the water footprint of your diet, meat is the place to cut back.

Water footprint per kilogram of crop and animal products

Vegetables: 322 litres/kg
Fruits: 962 litres/kg
Pulses: 4,065 litres/kg
Eggs: 3,265 litres/kg
Chicken: 4,325 litres/kg
Butter: 5,553 litres/kg
Pork: 5,988 litres/kg
Beef: 15,415 litres/kg

It takes nearly 15,500 litres of water to produce a kilo of beef, which is an astonishing 2,400 litres of water for one hamburger! One kilo of beef creates 27 kg of CO_2 emissions, compared to a kilo of lentils which creates 0.9 kg of CO_2. If, however, humans were to eat the kilo of grain themselves, that would be that. Along with not flying and driving less, going vegetarian is one of the very best things you can do for the Earth.

This is not a sermon – only a suggestion. You could eat less meat less often, purchasing only good quality, and still help the planet.

Treat Meat as a Treat

Remember those unusually long-lived populations who considered meat a rare luxury, rather than a staple of their daily diet? Cutting right back on meat is an unambiguously positive move for your health and for our over-populated planet.

You could start by reducing the amount of meat you eat on a weekly basis, maybe limiting it to weekends – even joining in the 'meat-free Mondays' movement can make a difference. You could also join in the global 'Veganuary' movement, where you eat vegan for the month of January – a challenging and healthy start to a new year: see *www. veganuary.com*. When you're consuming less meat overall, you can boost the quality, buying organic or locally reared produce instead of mass-market produce. Get to know your local butcher (and baker and candlestick maker!) in an effort to support your community. When the next horsemeat scandal breaks, you'll feel safe in the knowledge that you know where your meat is coming from.

You could even experiment with different sources of meat. The chef Richard Corrigan, who runs Corrigan's Mayfair, promotes the consumption of game such as venison, pheasant and grouse. 'What is more natural than game? It is wild, delicious meat that has come straight from the outdoors.' He attributes the rise in game consumption to a general concern about the provenance and traceability of food. There is also an increased awareness of the full range of wild produce in nature – if rabbit is OK, why not squirrel? – and a growing trend for nose-to-tail eating, which makes use of the whole animal. Game is also an economical option: in many local farmers' markets pigeon and rabbit are cheaper than other types of meat.

Vegan Revolution

Until recently, veganism was seen as worthy and laughably hippy, with a narrow repertoire of unappetising produce: mung beans, kale and nut roast. In the past few years, everything has changed. Meat-free Mondays have led to national Meat Free Weeks and even VegFests to celebrate the meat-free lifestyle. Vegetarian and vegan cafés and restaurants are springing up everywhere from Hackney to Los Angeles, with high-profile chefs, food writers and celebrities embracing the green-eating movement. Former US President Bill Clinton and Microsoft founder Bill Gates are both vegan. Ingredients are becoming more varied, expanding the options for experimental, tasty vegan and veggie cooking all the time. From vegan pizza to cupcakes to burgers, suddenly veganism doesn't seem so dreary after all.

Global numbers of vegetarians and vegans are hard to determine with accuracy. It's estimated that around two per cent of the UK population are vegetarian. According to the Vegan Society, there were around 150,000 vegans in 2014, which equates to around one in 400 people. The ratio goes up to roughly one in 150 in the US, according to the Vegetarian Resource Group, which puts the total figure at two million. Around the world there are many more semi- or part-time vegans.

This meat-free revolution has been driven by a combination of factors: health, animal welfare and environmental concerns. In the UK the majority of vegans cite ethical concerns, whereas in the US it tends to be more health-related, although ethical and health issues are closely linked.

As consumers, we're demanding more information and transparency over what goes into our food, especially following the scandals surrounding adulterated meat and other animal products. We're more aware of cruelty towards animals, the environmental toll and the unavoidable problem of sustainability: how the demands for mass meat consumption from a rising global population will be met.

Green Kitchen: an app for keen nutritionistas, packed with vegetarian recipes using ingredients straight from nature. You can sync the recipe timer with your smartphone to receive helpful notifications and reminders while you're cooking. All recipes are healthy, tasty and use minimal gluten, sugar and dairy.

If all this vegan talk is putting you off, remember: it doesn't have to be all or nothing. I'm semi-vegan and comfortable with that. This means that my diet is primarily based around plants, fruit, vegetables and grain, with the emphasis on natural and fresh. I don't eat meat, fish, seafood or eggs – but I won't freak out if something contains a bit of dairy: pesto, for example, or Greek salad with feta cheese.

Plenty of celebrities are fashionably opting for meat-reducing, or coming out as 'flexitarians' or 'vegan-curious'. They'll never give up their beloved bacon sandwiches, but they're increasingly happy to experiment with vegetarian cooking. High street stores and sandwich chains are offering a wider range of lunch and snack options with the vegan sign, which has helped to bring it into the mainstream. It only takes a few great vegetarian meals to make you see just how varied meat-free eating can be.

But What About Protein?

It's often thought that vegetarians and vegans are at risk of dietary deficiencies: iron, B vitamins and protein in particular. And it's assumed that meat is the best source of protein, especially for athletes and those with a very active lifestyle. You need protein for energy and to build muscles, right? That is emphatically not the case.

Look at nature: the most powerful animals on the planet – hippos, elephants, buffalo, for example – are vegan. Meat isn't the only source of strength. Protein is available from a wide range of non-animal sources, including nuts, seeds and plants. According to the Max Planck Institute for Nutritional Research, half of all amino acids are irreversibly damaged when heated to standard cooking temperatures – so eating raw or lightly steamed vegetables can actually provide more protein than cooked meat. As a vegan friend says: 'Why eat your protein second-hand, after it's been digested by the animal? Why not go straight to the source?'

🌿 Excellent bioavailable sources of iron include lentils, beans, pulses and green leafy vegetables.

Vitamin C is a nutritional 'helper' which increases the absorption of iron by up to two or three times, so it's a great idea to combine certain foods.

Super-charged food combinations include vitamin C-rich tomatoes with iron-rich brown lentils and spinach, or fruit such as kiwi, or a glass of orange juice, with iron-rich breakfast cereal.

All About Protein

'What is the difference between meat, dairy, soy, and vegan protein? Many people think that the usability of protein is a question of animal versus vegetable. However, even though animal protein is "more complete" than many vegetable proteins, it does not automatically make it better. For example, beef contains only about 20% usable protein. Spirulina and chlorella, on the other hand, average 75–80% usable protein – and these vegan options are just as complete and just as bioavailable. Combine the right yellow pea and rice protein and you can hit numbers approaching 85–90% usable protein... In the world of protein, nothing is necessarily what it first seems.' (www.nutribodyprotein.com)

Here are a couple of protein-rich concoctions which contain all the essential amino acids, ideal for muscle growth and healthy bones, as well as plenty of calcium and iron.

Vegan Protein Smoothie

Blend: ¼ pineapple, 2 apples, ½ ripe avocado, 1 medium banana (peeled), 1/4 teaspoon spirulina and 3 ice cubes

Contains: Essential fats, ALL essential amino acids, natural sugars, fibre, vitamins A, B, B6, C and E, riboflavin, iron, calcium, copper, phosphorus, zinc, boron, niacin, magnesium, folic acid and carotene.

Benefits? Packed with calcium, iron and essential amino acids, this is ideal for body builders, sporty types or anyone recovering after exercise. Zinc protects the liver and promotes bone formation, healthy immune system and wound healing.

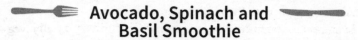

Avocado, Spinach and Basil Smoothie

Blend: 250 ml semi-skimmed milk (cow's milk or nut milk), handful of baby spinach leaves, 1 avocado, 1 chopped ripe banana (peeled), 2 tsp honey, juice of 1 lime, 1 tbsp of hemp, chia or any other seeds.

Contains: essential fats, pantothenic acid, fibre, vitamin K, copper, folate, vitamin B6, potassium, vitamin E and vitamin C.

Benefits: this is one seriously healthy breakfast smoothie! Packed with superfood ingredients for eye health, skin, hair, nails, and much more… It also makes a delicious salad (leave out the milk, honey and banana).

Don't Be a Vegan-bore

One of the decisions I made early on was never to verbalise my ethical reasons for vegetarianism (unless asked). Everyone in my family eats meat and fish, as do my partner and most of my friends. I don't lecture them about cruelty to animals or make them feel uncomfortable for their dietary habits. What could be more irritating than tucking into your Christmas dinner while someone mutters that 'meat is murder'?

> ❝ *I'm a vegetarian and I long for people to eat less meat, but the thing to do is not to go: "Eat! Less! Meat!" It's to say I am fit as a flea and I'm 63, I haven't eaten meat for 40 years. I never get diseases, I'm never ill, and I'm full of energy. So how's about that?* ❞
> **Joanna Lumley**

The truth is, simply being around a vegetarian makes many people feel implicitly rebuked. Hectoring others about giving up meat is a sure-fire way to turn them off. (The same goes for cycling, recycling and giving up smoking!) If I had any criticisms of the vegan movement – which on the whole I find a passionate and compassionate force for good – it would be that some of its followers lapse into militancy. You don't win people over by making them feel guilty.

Even some committed vegans admit that living a fully vegan lifestyle is not easy. Setting the bar so high is a risk. Attacking people for their much-loved leather boots, admonishing them for eating honey and demanding that they give up all non-vegan wine and beer are not ways to convert people, because these are not easy sacrifices to make. In the end, eating habits are an individual choice. The ideal is to find a primal balance: to minimise the damage our dietary choices have on the planet and to choose natural, sustainable sources of food.

The Health Perspective

Cutting out meat doesn't guarantee tip-top health or the perfect body: many vegetarians consume plenty of refined sugars and artificial ingredients. Nonetheless, studies show that vegetarians and vegans are slimmer, on average, and less likely to develop diabetes. Of course, they need to take care to eat a varied, balanced diet – but that applies to all of us, and can only be a good thing.

In late 2015, the World Health Organisation published a report which made headlines around the globe. Scientists analysed over 800 studies going back decades and concluded that processed meat should be added to a global ranking of carcinogenic substances, alongside cigarettes, arsenic and asbestos. Even as little as 50 g a day of products such as bacon, sausages, salami and ham is thought to increase the risk of colorectal cancers by 18 per cent. This is a surprisingly small amount: around an ounce and a half, or just two rashers of bacon. Other red meat, including beef and pork, was linked to higher risk of cancer, although not as much as processed meat.

So, does the WHO report vindicate that prediction at the start of this chapter, that 'eating meat will soon be as unacceptable as smoking'? Judging by current reactions, it seems unlikely. Opposition to the WHO's findings from meat-eaters was robust, to put it mildly, echoing responses in the mid-twentieth century, when the first anti-smoking health warnings began to emerge. Others talked of 'moderation in all things', including meat.

Only time will tell what the future holds for meat consumption. Nutritional science develops and social attitudes evolve. The ethical, health and environmental case for vegetarianism becomes ever more compelling. However we feel, whatever we eat, we cannot avoid these fundamental facts.

- We do not need to consume animals in order to access high-quality protein.

- Expecting to eat meat most days is environmentally unsustainable. Remember the water footprint of meat production? It takes 2,400 litres of water to produce a single hamburger. The growing meat consumption of our booming global population is exerting a huge toll on this already over-taxed planet.

- It's ethically indefensible. Terms like *free range* or *welfare-friendly* have been proved meaningless. No one wants to know what really goes on inside abattoirs. No one can deny that animals feel pain, just as humans do.

If we accept these facts, the question changes from *'Why are you a vegetarian?'* to *'Why do you eat meat?'*

Chapter 9
Primal and Seasonal

Living in tune with the changing seasons sounds like a nice idea, but in reality it can be challenging. You know how it goes: it's only November and you're battling through downpours in Cardiff, snowstorms in Chicago or sub-zero temperatures in Berlin. You haven't seen sunlight for weeks and you can't feel your toes. It can be hard to feel positive about winter when you're facing four or five months of this...

Spring and autumn tend to be a walk in the park (literally). In May it's easy to enjoy the carpets of daffodils, the budding of crocuses and bluebells, and the sense of renewal and optimism. In September you can read Keats's 'Ode to Autumn', marvel at the red and gold leaves, and eat Bramley apple pie.

Winter should be a time of snowflakes, sleighs and robin redbreasts – but that's just the fairy tale version. Too often winter is dark, damp and cold. It's no wonder that birds (and the super-rich) migrate to warmer climes over those long months.

One thing's for sure: the seasons haven't changed much since our primal ancestors walked the Earth. Whatever the significance of climatic fluctuations over the past decades and centuries (a contentious issue between scientists and sceptics), they would still have experienced the frosts of winter, the buds of spring and the heat of summer. Living *with* the primal seasons, instead of battling *against* them, is good for us. The American poet Mary Oliver has some beautiful lines about greeting each day:

66 *Hello, sun in my face. Hello you who made the morning and spread it over the fields...Watch, now, how I start the day in happiness, in kindness.* 99
Mary Oliver

> **What's Your Favourite Season – and Why?**
>
> **Eleni:** For me, spring is the best time of year. I'm originally from Greece, which has different weather patterns, but in the UK I love spring flowers, birds, the first days when you can go outside without a coat on.
>
> **Dan:** I'm weirdly affected by the seasons. Overall, I like summer best, but I get very depressed every year when August rolls around, and again in January. I don't know why but it happens like clockwork, mid-winter and mid-summer.
>
> **Susan:** I can't abide the heat! It's impossible to sleep or do anything except cower indoors with a cold flannel pressed to my brow. For me, the ideal weather is a crisp winter's day, going for a brisk walk, swathed in gorgeous scarves. Or some London rain.

Seasonal Affective Disorder

It's not surprising that Dan feels low in January: approximately two million people in the UK are thought to suffer from seasonal affective disorder (SAD), also known as winter depression.

These episodes of low mood, ranging from mild to severe, tend to occur at the same time each year, and are most acute during December, January and February. Sufferers often sleep more, become less active and find that they have little interest in life. The lack of light is thought to affect the function of the hypothalamus by interfering with certain brain chemicals, notably the hormones melatonin and serotonin (closely linked to sleep and mood). The reduced light also disrupts the body's circadian rhythm: the internal 24-hour clock which regulates sleep-wake cycles and other biological processes.

Huddling indoors away from the cold is a natural reaction to winter, but it only exacerbates seasonal affective disorder. Don't despair, though: there are ways to counteract this.

Lighten Up

Light therapy, sun lamps and special clocks during winter have all been shown to alleviate symptoms of SAD. They focus on one of the hardest characteristics of winter: the long, dark days. Special alarm clocks imitate sunrise, fooling your brain into thinking that it's time to wake up naturally, by turning brighter every minute. You can also buy strong light boxes to sit in front of at home or in the office: this artificial light supplies the energy that sunshine would normally provide.

The Sunshine Vitamin

Another winter hazard is a lack of vitamin D; this has several important functions in the body, such as regulating the amount of calcium and phosphates, which keep bones and teeth healthy. We derive most of our vitamin D from sunlight on the skin; it can also be found in oily fish (sardines, salmon and mackerel), eggs and some fortified breakfast cereals.

While most of us obtain adequate levels of vitamin D from a healthy diet and regular exposure to daylight, some groups (e.g. children under five, pregnant or breastfeeding women, those aged over 65 and those with darker skin) should take a supplement. If you're deficient, a daily supplement containing 10 micrograms (0.01 mg) of vitamin D is recommended. Do not take more than 25 micrograms (0.025 mg) a day, as it could be harmful.

Get Outside Every Day

Hiding indoors in overheated, artificially lit buildings is an understandable reaction, but will only make the situation worse. Getting outdoors is vital for anyone prone to SAD but also for general health. A brisk 20-minute walk at lunchtime, even in the weakest daylight, will make a difference. It will boost your vitamin D intake, activity levels and overall mood.

Winter Like a Scandi

When it comes to wintering in style, as usual, it's the people in seriously freezing countries who get it right. Winter far north of the equator can be brutal: with few hours of proper daylight, Norwegians, Finns, Danes, Icelanders and Swedes spend half of the year in what feels like perpetual night. Their 'dark season' can last from October through to late March, with temperatures routinely well below freezing.

However, even when the thermometer drops to −30°C, Nordics don't go into meltdown. The Danish have this beautifully primal concept of *hygge* which is all about being cosy, hunkering down and making your home a haven during the winter. *Hygge* focuses on inviting closeness with others, feeling open-hearted and alive, and paying attention to the present moment. *Hygge* is found in those small rituals you take pleasure in, whether it's lighting a scented candle or running a hot bath.

You're probably already hygging without realising it. Here are some examples of perfect *hygge* in action:

- sharing a home-cooked meal with friends and family
- lighting a fire on a rainy night and drawing close around the hearth
- brewing up real coffee for everyone at work and taking a break together
- wrapping up in wool blankets after a walk on the beach/around the park
- curling up in bed alone with a hot-water bottle and a great book.

Other Northern European countries have their own terms for *hygge*. The Dutch equivalent of cosiness is *gezelligheid*, which encompasses both the physical state of feeling snug and cosy, and the emotional state of being secure, 'held' and comforted. The German term *Gemütlichkeit* and the Finnish word *kodikas* carry similar connotations of homeliness, warmth, and well-being with friends and family. The English word 'cosy' itself comes from the Gaelic word *cosag*: a small hole you can creep into.

Dress for the Cold

Winter is also more manageable when you stay warm. Hence, the Norwegian saying: 'There is no bad weather, just bad clothing.'

Although UK temperatures may not dip as low as –30°C, good-quality winter clothing makes a real difference to your mood, health and the amount of time you can comfortably spend outdoors.

Layering clothes is crucial to preserving warmth: Norwegians wear between three and six layers, with wool and silk particularly recommended. Decent footwear is also important: ditch the high heels for work and wear a pair of sturdy, waterproof boots.

At home, the onesie is the ultimate *hygge* outfit. A sort of adult Babygro, onesies have become an unlikely trend in recent years, with even Chanel designing their own stylish all-in-ones. The idea is clearly that you climb into your onesie, zip it up and settle down on the sofa for the rest of winter.

> **Louise:** I realised that things were getting out of hand when my dread of winter started affecting me in September. Now I forbid myself from worrying about winter until at least October. I try to keep summer going as long as possible – I have holiday photos as my screensaver, and a bit of fake tan also helps!
>
> **Jane:** I deal with winter by treating myself. I buy nice things, even if it's just a new flavour of soup for lunch or a new scarf to give me a boost. I also plan weekends away to break up the monotony of those long dark months – in fact, I save holiday allowance specifically so I can get away during December and January.

Winter Getaways

I think Jane has the right approach: winter is an ideal time to catch up with friends you don't see enough, especially if they live in cosy country cottages. House guests are usually welcome if they arrive bearing chocolates, wine and flowers! Wherever you live, getting away for weekends is good for body and soul. What could be more primal than a long yomp through the fields or forests, followed by a hearty pub lunch beside a roaring fire?

If you don't have children, you can take advantage of out-of-season holiday deals. With all those spring bank holidays a distant memory, taking long weekends away is ideal. (Ever since the first *Bridget Jones* book came out, I prefer to call them 'mini-breaks' – preferably 'romantic mini-breaks'.) You might not reach winter sun on a weekend away, but you can definitely get to some fantastic places within Europe.

Hop on a Eurostar train and explore any of the German Christmas markets: Cologne, Frankfurt and Munich are wonderful. Amsterdam is a city of style these days, with wonderful art, fashion and food. I'd also recommend all the Belgian destinations, especially Antwerp, Ghent and Bruges, or the old-fashioned option: Paris.

Start planning your winter weekends, whether at home or abroad, and the cold weather will already seem more enticing!

Here are a couple of bonus primal points.

Taking the train is greener and more scenic (and often quicker) than flying. Not only do you avoid potential airport nightmares, but you also won't suffer jet lag.

Doing your Christmas shopping in Europe means you can find presents that aren't necessarily available in UK shops.

Eating Seasonally

Enjoying different produce at different times of the year is a fundamental aspect of living primally. When you're eating in tune with nature, you can't help but embrace the changing seasons. Even the end of the summer is a fruitful transition, with the abundance of natural produce that early autumn brings. Our ancestors had no choice but to eat whichever wild berries, root vegetables and nuts were available, depending on the time of year. With intensive farming, air freight and freezing, modern food production has all but erased these natural transitions, separating us further from the seasonal cycles of our primal ancestors.

It's not as easy as it sounds, and I'm no saint when it comes to eating seasonally. Like most people I've grown used to year-round delicacies:

why shouldn't I have purple sprouting broccoli in autumn, sweet potato in summer or cherries in winter? We may be able to access anything at any time, but have you noticed how much better seasonal produce tastes? Part of the joy of travel is tasting fresh produce from the local region: juicy grapes grown in the South of France, for example, or oranges in Seville, bananas in Ecuador or mangoes in Thailand.

The increasingly *non*-seasonal nature of our food culture is mostly our own fault: we've grown accustomed to having access to the same produce all year round. We'd be surprised not to be able to buy apples in summer, for example, just because it isn't the UK apple growing season. Instead we happily consume Pink Lady apples from Chile, Braeburns from New Zealand or Golden Delicious from the United States. According to the Department for Environment, Food and Rural Affairs, up to 70 per cent of apples bought in the UK have been imported.

The big supermarkets are also at fault, by catering to our constant demands. As the food writer Joanna Blythman points out: 'The supermarkets' obsession with stocking every fruit and vegetable grown on the planet, every day of the year, makes it hard to detect the ebb and flow of seasonal produce.'

It goes without saying that transporting fresh produce around the globe contributes to increased carbon emissions and exerts a heavy environmental toll. Local, seasonal food is more nutritious than produce which has travelled many thousands of air miles: it's a positive choice for the planet, positive for local farmers and food growers, and it's good for your health. Nature is extremely clever at providing the right nutrients for us at the right time of year.

> **Roger, 44:** During a few years when the downstairs flat was vacant, I planted up someone else's garden by stealth... Then a new tenant moved in. I eventually plucked up the courage to knock on her door and ask if she minded me growing a few carrots, and she was delighted! She worked long hours and had no time for gardening, and she was relieved someone was

dealing with "that wasteland". For several weeks I left thank you gifts from the garden at her back door but she didn't even pick them up, so I've stopped feeling guilty and I've stopped leaving vegetables! Now I've got a full-on market garden out there: potatoes, carrots, broccoli, runner beans, redcurrants, apricots, gooseberries, blackberries. Often I have more produce than I can consume – I've been known to turn up at my place of work (a further education college) bearing muddy bunches of radishes.

Foraging

If you can't grow your own, you can still pick your own. When you really look around, in the soil, on bushes and hedgerows, and up in the trees, you'll begin to see how tempting the countryside can be.

Foraging reconnects you with the land, with nature and with your food, and is satisfyingly primal. It's also healthy, sustainable and free. From mushrooms to nettles to crab apples, much of the produce that grows abundantly in nature can be used in the kitchen – no wonder they call the countryside 'nature's larder'. On a recent country walk I came upon a greengage tree on a public footpath, loaded down with tempting fruit. I filled my pockets with the ripest, and those under the tree (leaving plenty for others), and made a simple French-style compote when I got home – delicious with natural yogurt.

The food writer Hugh Fearnley-Whittingstall is a vocal advocate of foraging: 'Finding your own food seems to flick a primal switch, going back to when we were all hunter-gatherers, living incredibly close to the land... It only takes a little knowledge to make the most of each season.'

The British climate – despite being notoriously unreliable – is ideal for a wide range of seasonal, home-grown produce: we have enough sunshine to ripen fruit and nuts, and enough rain for crops and hedgerows. Farmers' markets, allotments and small garden patches are overflowing with nutritious tomatoes, aubergines, pumpkins, peppers, plums, apples and pears, and much more besides.

If you're imagining eating nothing but parsnips all winter long, fear not: seasonal fruit-and-veg consumption does not have to be dull! There are a million ways to spice up nature's larder: asparagus in butter, artichokes in vinaigrette, marinated aubergines, cherry tomatoes with mozzarella, basil and olive oil, roasted peppers, hand-cut potato wedges, spicy pumpkin soup, and so on – the list is endless.

Pick Your Own

If you don't have access to forests or meadows for foraging in the wild, picking your own is a great alternative. There are pick-your-own farms all over the UK.

With our renewed desire for greener, cleaner eating, lengthy waiting lists for local allotments and the growing popularity of urban gardening, the Pick Your Own movement has seen something of a rebirth. The nostalgia factor is strong: many of us remember happy childhood visits to pick-your-own farms, filling our baskets (and stomachs) with juicy strawberries, raspberries and blackberries.

Pick Your Own is also popular with adults. Compare the experience of buying overpriced, over-chilled – often flavourless – produce from a crowded supermarket with picking your own in the fresh air. Add to that the pleasure of knowing exactly what's in the food you're eating, eliminating transport miles and plastic packaging, and the sheer enjoyment of home cooking. You can take a picnic along, make a day of it, and return home with a carload (or bike basket-load) bursting with goodness.

A friend is a keen pick-your-owner, and I asked her what she liked about it:

" I love getting in touch with how food grows, seeing what it looks like before it's been tidied up, and touching the plants –

blueberries are easy to pick, while gooseberries won't let go of the goods without a struggle. Strawberries in the sun smell like strawberry jam – it's the smell of childhood. Ducking under the boughs of a heavily laden plum tree, or digging muddy carrots out of the ground with a fork.

Back home you have the pleasure of making dinner from food that you picked – it was in the ground this morning and will be in your stomach before bedtime! And if you make the fruit into jam, you get to enjoy the (literal) fruits of your labours long after that one day picking on the farm. It's also a fun way of being outdoors, feeling the fresh air on your skin, bending and stretching in ways that I don't in my office job – I'm not an exercise fan, so anything that has a practical purpose but also gets me moving is a winner for me.

Pick-your-own farms aren't the only ones opening up the countryside – you can explore farms with wildflower meadows and rare orchids, woodlands, and even aromatic sensory herb gardens. Some have rare breeds of animals, while others boast beautiful birds, bees and butterflies. With ventures such as Open Farm Sundays, farmers all over the country offer tours of nature trails, talks about their crops and even tastings. You can also learn about growing less familiar fruit and vegetables, and how to use them in your cooking.

Follow the PYO Rules

Some farmers have reported members of the public climbing over the gate and literally helping themselves – you can't wander onto another person's property and plunder their apple orchard! However, any trees or bramble bushes hanging over a footpath or right of way are yours for the picking.

Pick-your-own produce may feel more liberating than queuing at the supermarket, but you should still be mindful of the dos and don'ts.

Baskets, bags, punnets or wheelbarrows are usually provided, but some farms may charge a small amount, so take your own containers if allowed.

Be reasonable: you can pick enough to make jams and chutneys, or to fill the freezer, but don't take more than you need. It's easy to get carried away and end up with excessive amounts which will go to waste.

Harvest only the ripe fruit – unripe fruit should be left to ripen for other visitors.

Don't trample on plants and shrubs, and be careful not to damage the crops.

Pick only what you're supposed to: for instance, pumpkins but not their leaves (pulling them out damages the plant).

Apart from tasting small samples, don't eat the fruit while picking. Remember, a pick-your-own is not a free-for-all. These farms are mostly small, family-run businesses. Eating the produce instead of weighing and paying for it can lead to significant financial hardship. Respect that a PYO is somebody's livelihood.

Always pick up your litter.

And a few further tips…

Wear old clothes and shoes that you don't mind being stained; take gloves to protect yourself against nettles and brambles.

Whatever the weather, don't forget to apply suncream.

At home, wash your fruit and veg before eating and cooking with it.

Visit www.pickyourownfarms.org.uk to find your nearest farm, get tips on picking, and learn more about pickling and preserving fresh produce, bottling, freezing, how to make jams, pickles, and much more.

Right Time, Right Place

The truth is, most of us don't know what's growing when – a study by BBC *Good Food* magazine found that nine in ten adults could not identify the correct months when broad beans, blackberries or asparagus are in season... Could you?

Let's take a look at some of the fruit and vegetables available in the UK throughout the year.

Apples: January, February, October, November, December
Aubergines: May–October
Berries/currants (raspberries, strawberries, blackcurrants, redcurrants): June–September
Cherries: June, July, August
Pears: January, February, September–December
Purple sprouting broccoli: February, March
Rhubarb: March–September

Some produce, like winter and summer squash, artichoke, and beetroot are available pretty much all year round in the UK, and potatoes much of the year.

Other excellent resources online, including calendars showing the seasonality of meat, game, fish and seafood, can be found at:

www.eatseasonably.co.uk
www.vegsoc.org
www.bbcgoodfood.com/seasonal-calendar
www.whats-in-season.com.

Primal Cooking

If you're keen to use your primal foragings in the kitchen, a good place to start is by consulting Nigel Slater's recipes. I only discovered his cookbooks and cookery programmes recently, and he embodies everything that is wonderful about seasonal produce. He uses fresh ingredients, many of which come from his own enviably stocked London garden. He cooks in tune with the weather: refreshing, tangy salads in hot weather, for example, and hearty warming stews in winter.

Slater's relationship with food is also deeply primal: he touches it and smells it; he craves different flavours and textures, depending on his mood: searing hot lamb with cold cucumber yogurt dip, for example, or bread and butter pudding with creamy coconut milk and caramelised bananas.

His cooking is adventurous but not complicated, and doesn't rely on a million ingredients. It's based on simple, primal urges – for sweet and spicy, for childhood flavours, for comfort food – and who hasn't had those? His three volumes of *The Kitchen Diaries* are fantastic too, as much for the writing and food photography as for the recipes.

> **❝** *There are two spiritual dangers in not owning a farm.*
> *One is the danger of supposing that breakfast comes*
> *from the grocery, and the other that heat*
> *comes from the furnace.* **❞**
> **US ecologist Aldo Leopold**

Forgetting about farming is indeed dangerous. Losing touch with wild nature is bad for the planet and for our health. As we become increasingly removed from the process of growing and harvesting food, we endanger our relationship with the land. It's no wonder that many inner-city schoolchildren think that milk comes in cartons from the supermarket, rather than from cows. Many kids don't even understand that burgers, sausages and pre-sliced ham come from the processed body of an animal (and why should they, if they've never seen a living pig?).

And cows need pastures, and pastures need sunshine and soil and rain, and a delicate balance of fallowing and cultivating. Understanding nature's fragile equilibrium is ethically and educationally rewarding for children today, and for future generations. It will enrich their lives, and encourage them to exist more sustainably, more seasonally and, yes, more primally.

Look at the vast amounts of varied produce growing on our own little island – every month of the year there's something new to enjoy. When you start to experiment with seasonal food, imported produce flown halfway around the world begins to seem less appetising and less necessary. Suddenly, the experience isn't one of deprivation, but of abundance.

Nigel Slater describes his perfect blackberry and apple pie, with 'round, fat Bramley apples still wet from the grass... and tiny, sharp blackberries.' Like many of us, such primal flavours transport him instantly back to childhood. We may not boast Slater's culinary skills, but nothing beats picking, and then cooking, your very own blackberry and apple pie: juicy, sweet and perfectly in season. There is no need for imported winter cherries, when you could pick windfall apples and forage for hedgerow blackberries.

And this is what primal eating is all about: enjoying the natural produce of each season: looking forward to the first crop of baby new potatoes, for example, savouring the treats of winter and summer, spring and autumn, and finding primal pleasure in nature's larder. Not only is it good for you, and good for the environment, it's also a fantastic way to experiment with new flavours. Cooking with unfamiliar fruit and vegetables will widen your culinary range and boost your body's natural immunity. Healthy, green and clean: primal eating is a truly virtuous cycle.

Slow Food

As life has got faster, so has food. The Slow Food movement is a conscious rebellion against ready meals, on-the-go eating and fast food of all kinds. The movement originated in 1989 in Italy – the birthplace of long, lazy lunches – as a reaction against the gradual erosion of the country's traditional cuisine. These days, the philosophy of Slow Food is entering the mainstream, as indicated by the popularity of smallholdings, pick-your-own farms and farmers' markets. We're all about slowing down and pottering in our allotment, maybe feeding the chickens or making some plum jam.

Slow Food UK has some simple principles, all of which chime perfectly with primal cooking and eating.

Go Slow in Your Life

1. Buy whole ingredients. Cook them. Eat them.
2. Avoid processed stuff with long ingredient lists. Eat real food.
3. Grow some of your own food. Even if just on your windowsill.
4. Whenever possible, know the story behind the food you buy.
5. Buy local food; find out what is in season.
   (www.slowfood.org.uk)

Chapter 10
Primal Exercise

You should get sweaty and get hungry at least once a day.

Nothing is more primal than a really good sweat. Whether it's a morning run, a dance class or just everyday functional activity, getting out of breath and sweaty needs to be part of your daily life.

Everywhere you go, every move you make – travelling to work, walking the dog, cleaning the house, doing the shopping – is a quick and easy opportunity to raise your heart rate, rev up your metabolism and strengthen your muscles. You don't need to cut calories or enter an ultra-marathon: the aim is to be fit and strong, not super-skinny or rock-hard. Activity will leave you feeling recharged and refreshed, inside and out. Remember: your body is designed to move, get hungry and get sweaty *every single day*.

Mix It Up

Whatever you do, keep it varied. It's easy to fall into an exercise rut, whereby you spend half an hour on the treadmill on autopilot five days a week, because that's what you always do. Make a conscious effort to mix it up, alternating cardio with weights or with something a little more cerebral like yoga.

And listen to what your body feels like doing: if it's a beautiful day, how about a gentle jog along the seafront? If it's bad weather, how about vigorously clearing out the garage or garden shed? Remember that everything counts – lifting, bending, stretching, walking – as long as you're using your body.

Some of us are solo-exercisers, whereas others are team players. If you prefer exercising in a group, why not join a netball team (or start one)? Increase your agility with fast-moving activities such as badminton or squash, which demand quick, unpredictable movements. You could learn to dance: try ballet, Jazzercise, Zumba,

Salsa Jive, ballroom or whatever floats your boat. Thousands of UK gyms now participate in the 'class pass' scheme, where you pay an upfront fee and can try out different classes within a set period: anything from Pilates to spinning, strength training, barre or dance (see www.classpass.com). This is a great way of mixing it up and keeping your body, literally, on its toes.

> **James Duigan, personal trainer:** 'Anyone can run or lift weights, but the art is balancing everything so you do what your body needs, when it needs it. Ask yourself what you need from your workout that day – does it need to feel challenging, do you need to be energised, are you trying to clear your head? Using exercise in the way your body needs it is key to getting the right results.'

Exercise as we know it – as a formalised activity, in pursuit of the body beautiful, in mirrored studios – is a fairly recent invention. It's unlikely that your grandparents did regular workouts. However, movement has been intrinsic to human life since the dawn of mankind: movement *is* life. We know that moving improves mood, flexibility and cardiovascular health, and that not moving is bad for you. No surprise then that our increasingly sedentary, convenience-driven lifestyle is having a negative impact on overall levels of mental and physical well-being. While some people are doing plenty of exercise, sadly many are doing none at all.

In 2013, research conducted by the University of Bristol found that 80 per cent of UK adults were missing government targets of 30 minutes of moderate exercise at least five days a week. Out of more than a million adults surveyed, 46 per cent of people had not walked for leisure for 30 minutes continuously, 88 per cent had not been swimming and 90 per cent had not been to a gym in the previous weeks. And a 2015 study by the David Lloyd chain of fitness centres found that 48 per cent of respondents said that 'being fit and healthy was not an integral part of their lives'.

Everyday Movement

Being 'fit and healthy' really doesn't need to involve fitness centres. Primal exercise simply means moving your body more in everyday life – using what you have, and making it that little bit stronger, faster and fitter.

Your average caveman or woman's regular workout would have included pursuing deer, carrying water from the river, felling trees, hacking up firewood, carrying heavy rocks and running away from angry bears. All these sweat-inducing actions we now perform in gyms were originally part of staying safe, finding food, building shelters and keeping warm.

Domestic work was gruelling too: the food writer Bee Wilson reports that female skeletons from 10,000–20,000 years ago were routinely found with chronic arthritis, consistent with kneading, scrubbing and grinding activities. (Try using a pestle and mortar instead of a blender and you'll see why.)

For our grandparents and great-grandparents, too, daily life presented many opportunities for exertion. It wasn't formal exercise and it didn't need to be: before all our 'labour-saving devices', life itself was labour-intensive. Think of walking miles to school or to the factory (instead of driving), digging the allotment, carrying heavy shopping bags home (instead of ordering online), and wringing out the washing and hanging it on the line (instead of using machines). As a treat, they could look forward to going to the fairground or the beach, or dancing around a maypole (instead of watching Netflix on the sofa).

They didn't have gyms or spinning classes, but there was a hell of a lot more activity in people's lives. And this is why I'm in favour of ditching the gyms and the special equipment, and going more primal in your workouts. You know, *doing things*.

There's labour-saving and then there's downright lazy. These days you don't need to stand in the kitchen kneading dough to make bread, walk round the corner to the takeaway or even dial a number: you just tap the app, and pizza/curry/Chinese food will turn up at your door. Not surprising then that we're taking in more calories than we're burning off.

In June 2015 a study from Sweden hit the headlines, proclaiming that walking slowly in middle age could be linked to early death. Scientists from the Karolinksa Institutet analysed the data of nearly half a million UK adults, aged between 40 and 70, collected between 2006 and 2010. They were investigating which lifestyle questions could accurately predict the risk of death in the next five years.

Even without carrying out any physical examination, the researchers found that walking pace was a stronger predictor of death risk in both men and women than smoking habits and other lifestyle factors. It was concluded that slow walking could indicate serious underlying health conditions, such as shortness of breath, heart problems, disability and general ill health. Clearly, those who walk slowly are less likely to be vigorous and active, and more likely to engage in other sedentary behaviour.

Of course the Karolinska findings are open to interpretation, and don't conclusively prove cause and effect. Other studies have shown similar findings: walking pace and hand grip strength are indicators of overall health. It's a good reminder of the value of building moderate exertion into everyday life, especially from middle age onwards.

Green Therapy

Being outdoors – even without being active – is proven to be good for mind, body *and* soul. In 1984, Professor of Architecture Roger Ulrich reported that hospital patients appeared to recover more quickly from surgery in rooms with green views. Further scientific evidence backs up the health benefits of being in or near greenery.

- A view of nature can help the body to heal faster when we're unwell.

- A view of nature can help us to regain our focus when we're distracted.

- When we're stressed, images of a natural landscape can slow our heart rates, relax our muscles and promote a feeling of calm.

Natural daylight is a vital source of vitamin D and regulates the production of essential hormones, such as melatonin and serotonin, for healthy brains and sleep.

Exposure to natural daylight also keeps us alert and is a great mood booster.

Walk More

How did we get so addicted to our cars, buses and trains? In a recent tube strike, thousands of Londoners were complaining about having to walk miles to work. It's curious how outraged and inconvenienced we feel at having to trudge those few miles, when walking has been the dominant mode of getting from A to B throughout the history of the human race. In many countries it still is.

Think of the benefits of walking: a green, clean(ish) workout for free, which gets you exactly where you need to go. Walking can be faster than short journeys on public transport, especially in cities, and it's certainly more reliable. When you compare walking to stuffy journeys underground, endless bus queues or crowded commuter trains, it suddenly doesn't seem so bad after all.

There are numerous free apps which offer a range of workouts, from high-intensity Tabata to circuits to Pilates sessions. You can use them to track your daily activity and energy expenditure: just set your target – e.g. the recommended 10,000 steps a day – and they will tell you when you've reached it. Using apps to track your progress will keep you motivated and show how you've progressed. You can also create a personal profile and share with others around the world, if you like the idea of social networking and personal training all in one!

Treadmill vs Terrain?

Is all running equal? Experts usually recommend going for a run outdoors rather than running on a static treadmill. Here are a few of the reasons why running outside makes sense.

- **Satisfaction and results:** a 2004 study from Duke University found that treadmill runners ran more slowly, reported higher rated perceived exertion (RPE) and experienced lower satisfaction than those running outside. So, indoor running feels harder, delivers fewer benefits and is less enjoyable than outdoor running.

- **Biomechanics:** when you're running outside, you're adjusting to every slope, stone, incline or mound of grass, weaving around pedestrians, crossing roads, leaping over puddles, etc. You're in constant movement and this is great for the muscles and ligaments in the feet, for biomechanics, for overall balance and flexibility.

- **Repetitive:** running on a treadmill may cause repetitive strain injuries, such as shin splints, because the foot is falling continuously in the same way, in the same place. In outdoor terrain – whether on city streets or forest trails – the load and cushioning of the feet are constantly varied. In the same way, other changes in gait and stride have been observed in habitual treadmill runners, which don't occur when you're running in a more natural environment where your body can adapt to different gradients, acceleration, etc.

- Exercising outdoors has proven benefits for your mind as well as your body. Numerous research studies show that exercising outdoors reduces levels of cortisol, the hormone released when you're under pressure. It can reduce the brain's response to stress in the longer term, so you learn to handle the tough times better (Princeton University).

- Running outdoors is green, clean and free!

Personally, I prefer an invigorating 5K run along the canal over a treadmill session in a gym, staring at my own sweaty red face in the mirror. However, running indoors is still excellent exercise, so if you *are* a devoted gym-runner, that's fine too: treadmills have their place, especially in winter, and many successful athletes use them in their training. But as with all exercise, it's great to mix it up a bit. Pushing yourself out of your comfort zone helps to develop mental grit and physical stamina. Maybe alternate treadmill sessions with outdoor runs to keep your technique fresh and your enthusiasm stoked up.

More Reasons to Get Outdoors

Running isn't the only exercise you can take outside. The human body is designed to operate in motion, to lift and jump and run, rather than repeating static sets of specific exercises. And research shows that specially calibrated machines don't work our muscles as effectively as using our bodies. Just as we risk repetitive strain injuries when running in the same technique on treadmills, so we can get into a rut by repeating the same narrow sets of weights.

Of course, any workout is better than no workout at all, but where you can, go primal. A few alternative ideas which could occasionally replace the indoor gym are:

- climbing trees
- lunges, squats, press-ups and crunches in your local park
- sprint sessions between sets of bus stops
- infiltrating the playground (monkey bars are great)
- skipping and crawling.

As you can see, these aren't specifically primal exercises – sadly, there aren't many wild boars left to chase these days. But getting active outdoors, using park benches, grassy knolls and trees, makes all exercise feel elemental and fun. If you have an adventurous streak, plenty of sports centres and outdoors activity centres now have climbing walls, so you can try your very own primal scrambling. If you want to take it further, you could try bouldering or coasteering (with professional guidance, of course).

If you're into running and cycling, there are plenty of free apps. You can track your runs and bike rides using GPS, and also enter challenges against your own previous performance or other users'. If you're travelling, many apps will also show you popular local routes around the world.

Outdoor Gyms

If you're lucky, your local park may even have an outdoor gym. Exercising outside is common in other countries, from the ancient art of Zurkhaneh 3,000 years ago in Persia to Turnplatz outdoor gymnastics in Germany to morning Qigong in Beijing city parks. The modern forms of outdoor gyms were introduced in China in the run-up to their 2008 Olympic Games to encourage participation and raise levels of health and fitness, and the country now has over 37 million square feet of outdoor gymnasiums. In Shanghai participation is said to be as high as 45 per cent.

Outdoor gyms have begun to spring up in the UK, usually in the form of brightly coloured all-weather equipment such as pull-up bars, balancing beams, cross-training and stepping machines. They're often located in or near playgrounds to encourage parents to play at the same time as their children. The main provider, The Great Outdoor Gym Company, has installed over 400 such spaces in the UK since 2007, and there are many other companies.

Surveys have found that regular outdoor gym users experience an increase in their mental and physical well-being. There's a sense of variety and fun about working out in the open air (all the following quotes are from the Centre for Public Health report, Liverpool John Moores University, *Evaluating the Provision of Outdoor Gym Equipment*):

'... there was a grandad, the mum and the daughter on it. From about seven to about seventy, and everybody's going on it. I mean you wouldn't get people like that going to the gym, would you?' Users enjoyed trying out new things, playing with their friends and family, and having a laugh.

Outdoor equipment also fits in with people's daily routines: they're conveniently placed and don't require a special trip to the gym: 'Whether it's with the kids, the dog, or on my jogs, I'm in the parks all the time. So I could just hop on and do ten minutes or longer, however long I need...'

However, there is still some reluctance about exercising in public. Self-consciousness and embarrassment were the main reasons cited, as well as a lack of confidence in using unfamiliar equipment.

Functional Fitness

Functional fitness has its roots in physical rehabilitation, hence the emphasis on strengthening the body in practical ways. This is about using your body to perform as it was engineered to. Standing from a seated position, dragging, lifting and carrying are all simple functional moves.

Functional fitness can be basic or advanced, depending on your level of fitness. It's all about using your body's muscles. Remember: the message with muscles is use it or lose it. Middle age brings a natural slowing down of metabolism, weight gain and decline in strength, as well as a decrease in muscle mass. Through your 20s and 30s it's important to build, or at least maintain, muscle. Simple forms of functional fitness include squats, pull-ups, push-ups, jumps and dead lifts, all of which can be done at home or in the local park.

If you prefer to join a class rather than just bounding around your park, one of the latest – and most primal – forms of functional fitness is animal flow.

Animal Flow

Animal flow does pretty much what it says on the tin: it combines quadrupedal and ground-based movement, using all four limbs to crawl, climb, run and jump. You're moving opposing arms and legs in what's known as 'multi-planar, fluid, integrated movement' – look at the fluidity of how animals move across the ground. And you're using your own body-weight training to lift and move yourself.

This style of all-over workout is incredibly effective at building strength and working the muscles that traditional gym workouts don't reach. Other benefits include increased mobility, flexibility, stability, power, endurance, skill and neuromuscular co-ordination. Your body is not used to using all four limbs in this way, so it's mentally challenging too. It's also silly but incredible fun – dog, chimp or whatever animal you choose to channel – so you learn to shed inhibitions and live in the moment.

For all-over strength, fitness and flexibility, this is one of the best forms of primal exercise.

Use It or Lose It

Local spaces which aren't loved are likely to be lost. Whether it's an urban park or rural woodland, the green spaces around our homes should be valued and enjoyed. The more we're out there running or jumping around in our green spaces, the more we value them, and the more demand there will be to preserve and improve them. A park which is deserted and derelict will be easy to buy up and concrete over.

> **Naturalist Ray Mears calls the green belt:** 'Britain's greatest unofficial natural parks'. We need these spaces, and the birds and the trees need them too. So, cancel your gym membership, get out there and USE them!

It's widely acknowledged that green spaces are important for the population's health and well-being, but the upkeep of public parks is increasingly under threat due to local authority budget cuts. Parks funding in London has been reduced by 18 per cent since 2011, and the cuts could increase to 60 per cent by 2020. As well as the obvious stuff like mowing the grass and picking up litter, this funding is also essential for removing graffiti, fixing park benches, maintaining playgrounds and looking after trees.

Movements such as the Parks Alliance, Love Parks Week and Keep Britain Tidy campaign vigorously to stop UK parks becoming forgotten wastelands. From small patches of grass and shrubs to big recreational spaces, parks are our chance to go primal in the heart of our towns and cities. With rising property prices, growing populations and increasing housing demands, these oases of greenery are under threat from the concrete-over-everything urban jungle. Whether we volunteer, campaign or sign petitions for our parks, most of all: let's use them.

On Your Bike

This philosophy of use it or lose it, and the pressure of the crowd, is borne out by the recent cycling revolution. According to CTC, the UK's National Cycling Charity, cycle traffic has risen every year since 2008. In 2014, the total number of miles cycled in the UK was 3.25 billion, a growth of 3.8 per cent on 2013, and more than either motorcycle or bus miles travelled.

In the centre of many cities at rush hour you'll now see a mass of cyclists filling the roads. In London, for example, the number of journey stages made by cycle in 2013 went up to 0.6 million, a leap of 58.5 per cent from 1993. The number of people living in London who cycled to work more than doubled from 77,000 in 2001 to 155,000 in 2011, and Brighton, Bristol, Manchester, Newcastle and Sheffield have also seen substantial increases. In Cambridge, 29 per cent of working residents cycle-commute – a higher rate than that of any other local authority.

The UK may not have reached Dutch levels yet, but we're getting there – a new cycle superhighway has recently opened along the Victoria Embankment in central London: a glorious ride taking in St Paul's and the London Eye, all the way to Big Ben and the Houses of Parliament. This gives car drivers lots to complain about but, more importantly, gets the issue of safer cycling, bike lanes and cycle-friendly cities onto the public agenda in a big way. The more cyclists on the road, the safer it is for everyone to cycle.

A Breath of Fresh Air?

Even while resting, we inhale and exhale around 7–8 litres of air per minute – approximately 11,000 litres of air per day. We need oxygen for optimum brain functioning, clear thinking, glowing skin, good sleep and digestion. And of course, we breathe far more strenuously when we're active. So, while it's good to get primal and active outdoors, what are we actually inhaling?

Globally, the UN estimates that air pollution is responsible for around 3.3 million premature deaths a year. In the UK, levels of pollution are reaching – and far exceeding – dangerous levels: poor air quality is linked to life-shortening lung and heart conditions, breast cancer and diabetes, leading to 29,000 unnecessary deaths a year.

Nowhere is the problem more acute than in the capital. All 50 of the nation's dirtiest-air black spots are in London, and all are around roads where people live, work, go to school and shop, including Oxford Street, Park Lane and Knightsbridge. Levels of toxicity are up to three-and-a-half times the EU legal limit; nitrogen dioxide – a toxic gas linked to asthma, lung infections and other respiratory problems – has reached double the EU limit. It's estimated that vehicle emissions lead to around 7,500 deaths annually in the capital.

Surprising then that DEFRA says: 'Air quality has improved significantly in recent decades and we are investing heavily in measures across government to continue this, committing £2 billion since 2011 in green transport initiatives.'

The Clean Air Act (1956) was passed 60 years ago in response to London's Great Smog. While the Act undoubtedly brought a reduction in the large, smog-like visible soot particles, much of this pollution has been replaced by smaller, invisible emissions, also known as 'ultra-fine particles' (UFPs). These UFPs are arguably more deadly; we cannot see them and they pass easily inside buildings, in through car ventilation systems. They also pass easily into our lungs, our bloodstream and major organs, such as the brain and heart.

Anyone who lives in a busy urban area and exercises outdoors should be very concerned, because strenuous exercise and air pollution are a toxic combination. Heavy breathing and exertion mean that we inhale more deeply, increasing our exposure to these ultra-fine particles. Remember: these UFPs are the most damaging to our health (and face masks offer almost zero protection).

Tips to limit exposure to the worst of air pollution include:

- avoiding exercising near major roads and traffic black spots
- avoiding rush-hour peak pollution
- avoiding late afternoon exercise when ground-level ozone is at its highest.

These measures may reduce your exposure, but not that much. Clearly, action is needed on a much wider scale. Instead of improving filters, making particles smaller and switching from diesel to petrol, manufacturers need to reduce the overall amount of combustion aerosols in cities. We need to develop the technologies to replace polluting particles entirely. Meanwhile, go primal – use your body to get around. The more you can walk or cycle, and therefore the fewer cars and buses on our roads, the better. Another way to avoid pollution is to exercise indoors.

Sculpt and Tone Without Leaving Your House (and No Equipment Required!)

Chair pull

Start out lying underneath a strong chair, legs bent at a 90-degree angle and heels firmly rooted on the floor. Hold either side of the chair seat, palms facing inwards.

Push down into your heels as you use your arms to pull your body weight up, until your chest touches the underside of the chair seat (or as high as you can go).

Lower your body in a slow, controlled movement back down to the floor. Repeat eight to 12 times. Try not to arch your back.

This works your abdominal muscles and your core.

> **Basic Lunge**
>
> Keep your upper body straight, with your shoulders back and relaxed, and chin up; engage your core.
>
> Step forward with one leg, lowering your hips until both knees are bent at about a 90-degree angle.
>
> Make sure your front knee is directly above your ankle, not pushed out too far, and make sure that your other knee doesn't touch the floor.
>
> Keep the weight in your heels as you push back up to the starting position.
>
> Return to the starting position. Repeat 12–15 times on each side.
>
> This works your legs, boosts your balance and improves flexibility.

Focus

We often use exercise as an opportunity to zone out – to stare mindlessly at the screens in the gym or let our thoughts wander – but it could be time to sharpen up. Lifting your arms and legs up and down, or pounding the treadmill on autopilot, is boring for your mind and your body. Like other parts of your life, you can get stuck in an exercise rut. When your workout becomes just another task on the to-do list, or when it's not challenging you as it used to, it's time for a change.

Instead of zoning out, try really zoning in. Focus on each movement and squeeze the muscle you're working. This helps to recruit more muscle fibres and results in a much deeper workout. And don't forget the bus queue – an ideal time to tone those buttock muscles and work your pelvic floor muscles with a few Kegel exercises.

Time to Disconnect

While you're bringing that physical focus to each move, allow yourself to disconnect mentally. If you have a stressful job, you do a lot of thinking or you spend most of your time with other people, exercise is an opportunity to switch from brain work to body work.

This time away from colleagues and computers is ideal for self-reflection. Running, for example, can be a chance to sort things out in your head: after half an hour pounding the pavements, the park or the treadmill, seemingly intractable problems often grow a little clearer.

There's a man who swims in my local pool *wearing his iPod*. He's in the fast lane, leads looped around the back of his head and under his swimming cap, fully wired up. Sure, these devices are waterproof, but why on earth would you want that? What's wrong with silence or the soundtrack of splashing water? You often see people jogging and taking calls on their phone at the same time. It seems a shame that they can't give themselves half an hour to escape all that. The sense of freedom from the world – away from calls, emails, news updates, even music – is part of the joy of movement. Try a workout without gadgets: allow yourself to disconnect.

High Intensity Interval Training

High intensity interval training (HIIT) involves short, intense bursts of activity. If you're pressed for time, or get easily bored with repetitive routines, HIIT is a way of maximising your efforts into a compressed super-workout. For example, 20 minutes of a high-intensity workout can burn up to twice as many calories as the amount used on a longer, slower run.

Typically, HIIT is a mixture of speed and recovery: so, 60 seconds of exercise at your peak effort, followed by a recovery period of the same amount of time. This cycle of fast and slow should be repeated for around 20 minutes, three times a week.

Your peak effort is approximately 80–90 per cent of your maximum heart rate: you can work this out by subtracting your age from 220 or using a heart rate monitor. If you don't have a heart rate monitor, simply work on a rough effort scale of one to ten: if one is sitting in an armchair, and ten is 'I'm about to collapse', you should be aiming for eight or nine. If you're training at high intensity, you'll know!

It's a similar principle to running Fartlek (a Swedish word meaning 'speed play'): training with continuous variations of pace. So, fast sprints between lamp posts, for example, followed by a recovery jog, followed by another sprint, and so on – or a really fast cycle up a steep hill, followed by gently coasting back down. The HIIT principle can be applied to any form of exercise, on the cross-trainer, treadmill or spinning in the gym. When swimming, you can alternate fast lengths of front crawl with slower, recovery lengths of breast stroke.

Research shows that HIIT confers multiple health benefits, from improved heart function and blood glucose levels to reduction in joint pain, even among overweight and obese participants. (You're advised to see your doctor before starting any new exercise regime, especially if you have a pre-existing heart or other medical condition.) Numerous trials, including one from the American College of Sports Medicine, have shown that HIIT also continues to burn more calories *post*-workout than regular exercise. Best of all, HIIT workouts are usually rated as more enjoyable.

HIIT is also very primal. During those explosive bursts of activity, picture the woolly mammoth you're chasing with a spear; when lifting heavy weights, think of the boulders you need to shift for your new cave. Just like functional exercise, HIIT can be built into your daily routine – dance like a maniac when a great song comes on the radio, sprint all-out for the bus or run up and down the stairs!

Allow yourself to play and to rediscover the fun in exercise. HIIT is ideal when alternated with any form of cardio, such as running, cycling, aerobics or Zumba. Most of all, it's a great way of mixing it up, working all your muscle groups, maximising your time and effort, and avoiding boredom and burnout.

Seven-minute workout challenge: a high intensity interval training programme devised by experts which guides you through exactly what to do and for how long. It's a set of 12 exercises, each performed for 20 seconds, with a rest of 10 seconds in between. If you're seriously short of time but willing to put in the hard work, this level of HIIT will rev up your metabolism and keep it going even after you stop.

Fasted Training

This is also known as 'train low, compete high'. Contrary to the traditional technique of carb-loading before exercise, new research shows that working out on an empty stomach can be an effective way to boost performance and burn fat. A 2015 study in the *British Journal of Nutrition* found that when subjects were fasted during morning cardio, they burned 20 per cent more fat than when they had a meal beforehand.

So how does it work? Fasted training has been shown to enhance the mitochondrial adaptations that occur in aerobic training. This improves the body's ability to use fat as a fuel source during exercise, sparing muscle glycogen for when it is most needed, when exertion increases. It's thought that when the body learns to exert itself without any food, it gets better at performing when it does have fuel in the tank. It can be an effective strategy for relatively short training periods, anything up to 60 minutes. (NB this is not recommended for high-intensity activities or longer races, which require adequate fuel.)

The most practical way to incorporate fasted training into your routine is to train in the morning before having breakfast. Hydration is essential, so you should always drink plenty of water. You should also refuel following exercise: this is not about cutting overall calories, but a strategic training method whereby carbohydrate fuelling is completed *after* training rather than before.

Post-workout Repair

Eating protein and carbs following exercise will help to repair muscle and tissue damage, build lean muscle, and boost your metabolism.

Protein: excellent sources include pulses, eggs, tofu, fish, chicken, turkey, nuts and seeds.

Carbohydrates: brown rice, sweet potatoes, quinoa, sourdough or rye bread and vegetables

Fats: essential for ensuring that vitamins and minerals in your diet are properly absorbed. Avocado, healthy oils and fish are good sources of fats and carnitine, which supplies energy to exercising muscles.

Antioxidants

In vigorous exercise, oxygen consumption can be up to ten times as high as normal. This creates free radicals, or so-called 'oxidative stress', which need to be mopped up. This is the role of antioxidants. They help to prevent muscular fatigue, inflammation and cell damage, which occur during and after exercise. Without antioxidants in our diet, we increase our susceptibility to cancer cells and premature aging.

Fresh fruit and vegetables are an abundant source of antioxidants. Specifically:

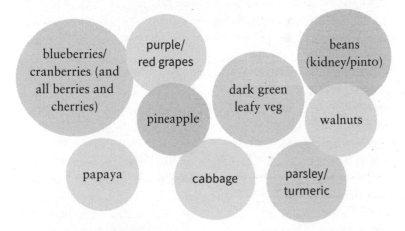

blueberries/cranberries (and all berries and cherries)

purple/red grapes

beans (kidney/pinto)

dark green leafy veg

pineapple

walnuts

papaya

cabbage

parsley/turmeric

A Weighty Issue

It's easy to assume that cardiovascular exercise is enough to stay in shape. Well, forget the stereotype of beefy men pumping iron in the gym: weightlifting is important for everyone, male or female, young and especially old. As we age, our muscle mass declines, leading to a less firm shape, and lifting weights improves muscle tone and definition. It also helps to maintain a healthy body weight and increases calorie-burning lean tissue. Remember: lean mass (muscle and bone) is metabolically more active than fat – or hungrier for energy – so you'll automatically use more energy even after you finish exercising.

Weights are also vital for combatting visceral fat – the invisible, often dangerous, fat wrapped around organs deep inside the body – and unhealthy belly fat.

In addition, muscles act as the store cupboards for carbohydrates, so the more muscle you have, the more carbohydrate you can store there as glycogen, readily available for energy, without converting it to fat.

Go Hard

Researchers have found that intense exercise is the most effective way to target visceral fat. A study published in the journal *Medicine & Science in Sports & Exercise* compared the reduction of visceral (internal) fat in people training at different intensities. Some participants continued with their regular exercise and others switched to high intensity, each for five days a week. The training time was adjusted for each session so that all the participants burned off the same number of calories. Only those who trained at a high intensity saw significant reductions in their visceral fat. Intense exercise and HIIT have also been shown to shock the body into releasing fat, as well as improving insulin resistance and increasing metabolic rate.

Eating for Strength

Social media is awash with #fitnotthin and #strongnotskinny hashtags: it seems that thin is out and strong is back. After years of unrealistic and unhealthy expectations on women's bodies, fitness and strength are the new goals.

Of course, the labelling of women as 'real', 'curvy', 'skinny' or 'waiflike' is still irritating as hell – guess what? We're all 'real' and our bodies are not fashion items to be deemed 'in' or 'out' with the changing of the seasons. But on the whole, the focus on genuine health and fitness has to be preferable to the obsession with losing kilos, inches, getting thinner, lighter (sadder). After all, in order to be active and energetic, you have to be well nourished. It matters that women can EAT and have energy, and still be beautiful! So let's embrace it! A glass of kale juice isn't going to replenish your body, nourish your skin or fuel your brain, however healthy it may be. Work out without enough protein in your system and you'll lose muscle, not gain it.

Figures such as Rihanna, Jennifer Lopez and Kim Kardashian are visible proof of the fact that you no longer have to be thin to be winning.

Strong and Happy

If you haven't already seen it, take a look at Sport England's *This Girl Can* – an inspiring short film which celebrates girls and women in all their diversity, different shapes, sizes, colours and ages. It's refreshing to see women getting out there, being active and enjoying their bodies for what they can do, rather than how they look.

I showed this film to a group of ten-year-olds when giving a talk on body image at a girls' school – they were so fired up by it that they made me play it three times over!

As well as giving your body tone and definition, muscle is important for health. Weightlifting three times a week can increase bone density by up to 19 per cent. This is particularly important for women, who are at risk of thinning bones as oestrogen declines with age (especially post-menopause). Weightlifting can also reduce the risk of stroke by 40 per cent and heart attack by 15 per cent, according to the University of Michigan.

If you're not a member of a gym, you can easily incorporate weights into your daily routine. Buy some free weights, kettlebells or dumbbells to use at home: leave them by the TV and get lifting during the ad breaks. If you're new to weights, you can start with as little as 1 kg and build up steadily. Sets of weights are cheap and easily available from any sports store or online. Alternatively, buy hand and ankle weights and wear them while walking the dog.

It doesn't need to be daunting: start with one or two sessions of weights a week, in between cardio activity such as walking or running, with eight to ten repetitions of each exercise. Stay safe and listen to your body. You shouldn't be straining to lift – you want to get toned not injured. If you start to love it, and want to do more, CrossFit weightlifting classes are intense and challenging.

Kettlebells

With their slightly daunting 'Iron Man' appearance, kettlebells can be off-putting. Think again! First developed by Russian farmers in the eighteenth century to measure out crops, these odd-shaped weights help to improve cardiovascular functioning, strength and flexibility, and to burn fat. You can lift, hold or swing them to build both upper- and lower-body strength. They take some getting used to, but when you get the 'swing' right, you won't look back!

Once you start, you'll see many opportunities to work those muscles: lugging heavy bags of shopping home counts, as does lifting bottles of water or tins while waiting for the kettle to boil, or carrying your kids around. If you are a member of a gym, ask one of the trainers to help you select the correct weights and use the equipment safely.

Wild Swimming

> 66 In the past 10–15 years there's been a resurgence of people going back to rivers and lakes and ponds. There is definitely a movement towards getting back to the great outdoors. 99
> **Caitlin Davies, author of** Downstream

In 2011, the comedian David Walliams swam 140 miles of the River Thames to raise money for charity. Many of us were filled with admiration, if not for the physical feat, for the sheer courage: the river is truly filthy, with around 39 million cubic metres of sewage pumped into it every year. But rest assured: wild swimming doesn't need to be quite so grim!

I've taken part in Christmas Day swims at various London lidos. These are in the 'so shocking it's amazing' category of life experiences. With air temperatures below freezing, and water temperatures not feeling much higher, it's so cold it makes your teeth ache – but also completely exhilarating.

Water is essential to all living organisms: between 60–70 per cent of the human body is made up of water (the brain and heart are composed of 73 per cent water, and the lungs are about 83 per cent water). Floating inside our mother's womb is our first experience of life. This may explain why water is mentally and physically therapeutic.

Swim to stay young! It won't literally turn back time, but swimming has been shown to cut the risk of dying early by nearly 50 per cent. According to a study carried out by Dr Steven Blair at the University of South Carolina, swimmers have the lowest death rate. This was a longitudinal study, carried out over 32 years. The research team followed 40,000 men, ranging from 20 to 90 years old and discovered that those who swam had a 50 per cent lower death rate than runners, walkers or men who got no exercise.

Whether it's in an outdoor lido, a traditional indoor pool, a lake, river or pond, swimming has many benefits. It's a complete cardiovascular conditioning and all-over aerobic exercise. It's anti-ageing, cuts the risk of diabetes and obesity, and improves flexibility. Swimming is also low-impact, ideal for those with arthritic or musculoskeletal conditions, as it avoids stress on the joints.

Swimming is routinely recommended in pregnancy, with benefits for both the mother and the unborn baby. According to a study from the University of Maryland: 'Water exercises involve no impact, overheating is unlikely, and swimming face down promotes optimum blood flow to the uterus.'

> **Kathryn, 67:** I've had rheumatoid arthritis for the past 30 years. During a bad flare-up my joints are so painful that I can barely walk. Swimming has been a lifesaver during the worst times, because it supports me and keeps my limbs moving. I call it my water therapy.
>
> **Polly, 34:** I'm eight months pregnant and still swimming every day. Moving around at this stage is pretty cumbersome, as my bump is huge, so getting into the pool is such a relief. It keeps me flexible and strong, and also helps me sleep. I'm even thinking of having a water birth.

Here are a few more reasons why swimming belongs in your life.

- Swimmers have been shown to experience significantly less tension, depression and anger after exercising than before. Rhythmic and aerobic forms of exercise such as swimming improve psychological well-being. Indoor lane swimming is calming and restorative; a freezing outdoor dip is invigorating and kick-starts all your body systems.

- Different swimming strokes challenge different muscles within the body. You can alternate between breast stroke and front crawl – even butterfly if you're feeling ambitious. (Warning: butterfly usually ends badly!)

- Water is about 800 times denser than air so you can work harder and burn more calories in a pool than out of it.

- The pressure of water causes a shift of blood volume from the periphery of the body to the thorax. This increases venal pressure and so leads to a decrease in heart rate of up to 20 bpm. In the pool, you can do the same intensity of exercise at a lower heart rate.

Safety Tips for Wild Swimming

Wild swimming is not for beginners: tides can be strong and unpredictable.

Check local rules and regulations, and always swim with others.

Wearing a brightly coloured swimming cap helps to keep you visible. It's also advisable to have someone watching on shore.

It may feel adventurous, but remember that some open water is polluted, dangerous and even illegal to swim in. You can't just go breaking into reservoirs, basins or industrial sites.

Never drink and swim (after a boozy summer picnic, this is very risky).

Wear adequate kit for the water conditions.

Avoid icy-cold temperatures if you have a heart condition (or similar medical issue).

For all these precautions, swimming outdoors is still a wonderful activity. For those lucky people who live near crystal-clear rivers or lakes, or within walking distance of the sea – I am very jealous! But it's surprising (even in our crammed-in, stressed-out cities) to discover how many undiscovered corners of watery tranquillity there are. Swimming in wild, open water is deeply primal and reconnects us with nature.

Don't forget the ocean: sunshine to restore you, salt water to heal you, waves to gently buffet you and sand to give you an all-over body exfoliation. Whether you live close to the coast or you're on holiday at the seaside, grab every opportunity to take to the high seas.

Kate Rew, founder of the Outdoor Swimming Society says: 'It's important with the heat and the stress of the city around you, to find a way of escape. Just get in the water. That entire world, which we've artificially created for ourselves, vanishes. I love that ability of swimming to give you a weekend within an hour.'

Find Out More
www.secretadventures.org
www.londonsroyaldocks.com
www.totallythames.org/events
www.outdoorswimmingsociety.com
www.swimtrek.com

White and Brown Fat

Humans have several different types of fat. First of all, the large deposits of energy-storing white fat. This is the stubborn podgy fat which settles around hips and stomach, and which we tend to pile on by eating unhealthy food and not exercising. Then there are smaller pockets of brown fat, whose main purpose is to keep us warm. Indeed, this brown fat produces 300 times more heat than any other organ in the body, and so burns through calories very quickly. Brown fat is plentiful in babies but drops to almost zero in adults.

Research in recent years (from, among others, the University of California) has found that exposure to the cold activates this special kind of 'good' brown fat. According to Stephan Guyenet, an obesity researcher at the University of Washington, 'Brown fat works like an internal fireplace, pulling glucose from the blood and from white fat stores in order to keep up the body's core temperature.' Put simply, brown fat burns white fat.

When the temperature drops, it's tempting to stay indoors with the heating turned up. Going outside to run, cycle or swim might seem uninviting, but it could be the smartest move you make all winter. Exercising outdoors in low temperatures can improve your performance, stamina and weight loss. And since your body is working harder to stay warm in the chill, you can even get away with brief, more focused sessions: a short, sharp sprint (or an icy dip) could be as effective as a long run, based on the principles of high intensity interval training. This is a fantastic way to start your day and helps to combat the winter blues which can set in during the dark months.

The heart is forced to work harder to distribute blood throughout the body in colder temperatures, so wearing the right kit is important. Layer up with thin, breathable tops which you can remove as your body temperature increases. When it's extremely cold, protecting your extremities is essential: wear a lightweight hat and gloves.

Cold muscles can be stiff, so it's particularly important to warm up properly in cool weather: start running more slowly than usual to ease yourself in. Cold weather exercise is not recommended for those who are overweight or very unfit, or those with heart conditions, as frigid temperatures can cause blood vessels to constrict, raise blood pressure and increase strain on the heart.

Dial It Down

The brown fat principle is applicable in everyday life, too: keeping temperatures cool at home and in the office will help to activate 'good' calorie-burning brown fat. Dutch researchers at Maastricht University Medical Center found that frequent exposure to mild cold temperatures sped up the body's metabolism, thereby boosting energy expenditure.

Scientists have also investigated the effect of sleeping at cooler temperatures on metabolism. They found that the amount of brown fat doubled during the weeks when participants slept at lowest temperatures, effectively speeding up their metabolisms. Acclimatising to cold temperatures can also help to train your body to burn more fat overall, and can help with healing. Many elite athletes use ice chambers as part of their training and recovery regime, as they stimulate increased blood supply.

If our bodies respond to the cold by speeding up our metabolism – a sort of inner central heating – it stands to reason that we shouldn't keep ourselves too warm. Central heating not only dehydrates the skin, and uses precious environmental resources, but also prevents the good brown fat from doing its job. How warm is too warm? Well, if you're walking around your house in T-shirt and shorts all winter, that's wrong. Turn down the heat, go for a run in the cold, cuddle up to a friend/lover or put on a jumper. Turning down the thermostat is good for the planet and good for your body too.

All About the Foot

Perhaps the most important part of your body on this primal journey is your foot. Considering that feet walk around 7,500 steps a day – or well over 100,000 miles over a lifetime – and that they carry our entire body weight, balance us, transport us, support us and ground us, we give our feet surprisingly little thought. It's the part of the body we take least care of, allowing them to get hard and gnarled, often even cramming them into tortuously high heels. Our feet are, quite literally, the foundations of everything we do. Why do we take them for granted?

With 66 joints, 214 ligaments and 38 muscles, and 25 per cent of the body's bones, the human foot is a work of engineering genius. And remember: when these anatomical miracles first formed, they weren't intended to function in shoes. The bare human foot is about as primal as it gets.

Going barefoot at home, in the office (under your desk), in the garden and wherever else you can will improve your balance, strength, circulation and posture – and make your feet feel great. Wear thick socks if the floor is cold. Alternate between different shoes every day, if possible, to keep all your bones, muscles and ligaments flexible, and give yourself time off high heels. Treat your feet to the attention they deserve. Try the occasional pampering scrub, massage those aching toes and arches, and finish off with some cooling lotion.

Barefoot Running

> 66 *My own prescription for health is less paperwork and more running barefoot through the grass.* 99
> **Leslie Grimutter**

Humans have been at it for thousands of years – but now barefoot running is officially a thing. Advocates claim that footwear constricts our feet and inhibits natural movement, leaving us prone to injuries, pain and postural problems. It all sounds awesomely primal, but choose your environment carefully (and watch your step). I've seen people barefoot running through the centre of London, over broken glass, jagged paving stones, dog excrement and goodness knows what else…

This is one fitness trend it's best to save for a mossy forest trail or sandy beach; even if you don't mind the soles of your feet becoming black with filth, you could sustain a serious injury. Researchers at Brigham Young University found that runners who made the switch from normal trainers to barefoot shoes too quickly suffered an increased risk of injury to bones in the foot, including possible stress fractures, pulled calf muscles and Achilles tendonitis, with some patients laid up for several months. There is also the risk of serious cuts and infection when running on uneven surfaces, especially those littered with the usual city-centre hazards.

Instead of going completely bare, try minimalist coverage. Barefoot running shoes act like a glove for the feet and are designed to protect them from glass and other hazards on the ground. And remember that although primal man was not designed to wear shoes, as modern humans we've been wearing them all our lives. Our feet are softies, in evolutionary terms, unnaturally reliant on overly cushioned trainers. In order to adjust to new stresses and pressures on the small bones and muscles, make the transition gradually. If you're keen to adopt a more primal style of running but don't want to risk injury (or, like me, find the five-toed foot gloves rather creepy!), try the thinner, more responsive breed of trainers, such as Nike Frees. They're slim and specially designed to support the natural motion of a runner's feet, but have fewer bouncy layers of air of the old-style trainers.

Mindful Walking

Walking has numerous physical benefits, especially if you're not ready for vigorous activity or prefer your exercise to be low-impact. It's also excellent for mental well-being.

Whether you're walking alone, deep in thought, or with someone else, it offers an opportunity to work through problems or broach difficult topics. People tend to talk more openly and personally when walking: being in step together promotes a kind of harmony and understanding. Walking avoids the pressure of a face-to-face confrontation, and gets the mind and body working in harmony. It's rare to have a blazing row or 'storm out' when walking together, after all!

A walk can happen anywhere…

- When you're travelling, it's the best way to see the sights.

- When you're working, it gets you away from your desk.

- It gets you from A to B without the hassle of public transport.

- A good walk can take place in the busiest city streets or the most remote beaches and mountains.

- There have even been recent trials in 'walking meetings' – like standing desks, these are a nice idea, but who knows if they will catch on!

- As an added bonus, getting outside for a walk boosts essential levels of vitamin D.

How Vitamin D Guards Against Weight Gain

Researchers at Aberdeen University studied 3,100 women in the north-east of Scotland in 2008. They found that the bodies of women who were clinically obese contained ten per cent less vitamin D than those of a healthy weight. Dr Helen Macdonald, who led the survey, says: 'Lack of sunlight interferes with the hormone leptin which tells our brain when our stomach is full, so we feel compelled to eat more.'

In addition, when deprived of sunlight, the pituitary gland in the brain also lacks stimulation and our brain responds by thinking it is in the depths of winter. This makes us more likely to adopt 'survival tactics' such as staying inside, exercising less and eating whatever is available.

Primal Core

At the heart of primal fitness is a strong body. This is not about trying to achieve Iron-Man levels of strength, or an aesthetically 'perfect' physique; it means being active and energetic, comfortable and confident with your body, healthy and happy in yourself. Daily life offers endless opportunities to move, lift, lunge, stretch, bend, run, jump, raise your heartbeat and break a sweat. The more regularly you recruit your muscles, in as many varied ways as possible, the more core strength and flexibility you naturally build.

Your core is a complex series of muscles which go far beyond the abs or glutes. It has three-dimensional depth and functional movement in all three planes of motion. The core muscles lie in and around the torso, including the stomach and pelvic floor muscles, and mid- to lower back. Many of the muscles are hidden beneath the exterior musculature that people typically train. The deeper muscles include the transverse (upper and lower) abdominals, multifidus, diaphragm, pelvic floor, and many others. Here are five essential things that your core gives you:

- strength

- endurance

- flexibility

- motor control

- function.

As we've seen, our primal ancestors were strong through necessity, not from repeating narrow sets of exercises in gyms. They relied on their bodies for everything, from food to transport to ultimate survival. Incorporating similar principles of functional fitness into our own primal attitude helps us to build a solid core.

A strong body doesn't just look good; it's also more resilient and less prone to disease or infection. Core stability supports the spine and surrounding musculature to ensure good posture. Research has shown that athletes with higher core stability have a lower risk of injury. A strong core also protects your inner organs, helps the body to recover more quickly and even burns calories more efficiently. Moreover, core muscles are crucial in everyday actions such as staying continent, emptying the bowels, speaking, singing and even breathing! You use your core, often without realising, in almost every physical movement.

The most effective way to work your core is to focus on movements based on your own body weight (as opposed to external equipment). You're effectively playing gravity against your own weight to build stamina and balance. Instead of obsessing over the washboard stomach or chiselled abs, concentrate on strengthening the muscles deep within! Here are some simple core-strengtheners to work into your daily routine:

- plank and side-plank
- abdominal crunches
- pull-ups on bars (or playing on money bars)
- bridge
- bicycle kicks.

Try lower body exercises such as dead-lifts, lunges and lateral band walks. These will engage the glutes, and tone your thigh and buttock muscles. Squats, which you can easily do at home or in the park, engage the muscles deep in your back and stomach, whittling your waist for a sculpted shape.

If you prefer classes, Pilates, yoga and ballet are also fantastic ways to target the core and strengthen your body from within.

Primal exercise should really be thought of as primal movement, because it's exactly what your body was designed to do. Whether it's walking the dog, running for the bus, carrying the shopping bags or a more strenuous form of workout, your body will thank you for moving every day. If it raises your heart rate and gets you sweaty, so much the better! Never miss an opportunity to leap, sprint, bend, twist and turn: enjoy your body's full range of flexibility and strength. Like the rest of your primal journey, primal movement is green and clean: good for you and good for the environment. There is no downside: the more you move, the better you feel.

Just as we should value our green spaces, urban parks and hidden corners of tranquility, we should appreciate our bodies: remember, the same use it or lose it principle applies. Every form of movement counts, and there's something for everyone: if you don't like gyms, do a yoga session online; if you can't swim, take to two wheels; if you're feeling adventurous, try a rock climbing or ballroom dancing class. If you just don't like formal exercise, go for a long walk, tidy up the garden or lift some weights while watching TV. Whatever your age, body shape or level of fitness, simply using those muscles will make you happier and healthier, stronger and more supple.

Tuning into your body's natural impulse to move is transformative. Just as primal eating encourages you to listen to your appetite, so primal exercise increases awareness of your physical health. It's also great for your mental well-being: exercising, alone or with others, is the perfect time to sort out emotions or troubles. Primal exercise can be hard work, in a good way, but it should never feel punitive. Enjoy it! Don't work out because you hate your body. Work out because you love it.

Chapter 11
Primal Beauty

A positive, accepting attitude to your body is at the heart of primal beauty: this is where it starts. Being healthy and happy outshines any number, whether that's the number on your birth certificate or the number on your bathroom scales. Appreciate your perfect bits, smile at your imperfect bits and to hell with the rest!

What Does Beauty Mean to You?

Was there a time in your life when you felt beautiful? Maybe the first time you fell in love, when you learned to dance or took up a new sport. Respecting your body for what it does as well as how it looks is a powerful act; for women especially, it can be a game-changer. Too often we compare ourselves with impossible 'beauty' standards, and criticise ourselves when we fall short. Primal beauty means learning to value our well-functioning bodies and the simple miracle of being alive.

Reject the Stereotypes

With the resurgence of feminism, we're gradually moving away from rules and expectations about how women should *behave*. However, there are still plenty of idealised notions of how women should *look*. The traditional beauty stereotypes are fairly narrow: slim, blonde and pretty, tall, dark and sexy, or some combination of the two. Being young helps, as does being thin. But who invented these rules, and who says you have to conform? Primal beauty is about finding the confidence to reject these stereotypes, celebrate your own unique look, and express your personality and appearance however you want.

Primal beauty also means inventing your own version of beautiful, which transcends fads or fashions, make-up or Manolos. It's that kind of beauty you feel halfway through a summer holiday, when you're relaxed and sun-kissed, wandering around with bare skin and beachy hair, glowing with health, happiness and tropical fruit smoothies. Gorging on fresh watermelon and huge salads, you can't imagine eating comfort food or wearing opaque winter tights ever again.

Hold On To the Glow

For most of us the hippy beauty fades as fast as the suntan, but there's something here worth holding on to. The reason we feel beautiful on that precious fortnight in Ibiza or Barbados is that we've left our cares behind. Far away from the stresses of everyday life, the train commute, the relentless emails or the office politics and the morning alarm, we sleep more and worry less. The mega-infusion of vitamin D gives our skin a glow which is impossible to fake, and hot weather naturally encourages us to consume lighter, fresher food.

You know the saying: beauty is skin-deep. In fact, it goes far deeper than that. True beauty has far more to do with what's going on inside, and you can help it to shine through by thinking positively, eating well, sleeping deeply and living kindly. Think about those transformative moments in life, and how radiant they make us: every bride looks beautiful on her wedding day, as does every mother cradling her newborn. Inner joy shines out: that's what we're aiming for with primal beauty.

Chuck Out the Scales

The first step is to debunk the tired old message that thin is beautiful.

Most women, if they're honest, would put targets such as 'losing weight', 'eating less' or 'getting thin' at the top of their mental checklist. In fact, when you actually talk to women whose weight has fluctuated significantly, the thinnest times have not coincided with the happiest times. Quite the opposite: often their leanest times have been the most lonely and miserable in their lives.

This makes sense: depriving yourself of good nutrition is a wretched experience. Genuine beauty does not depend on being thin. Every part of your body suffers when you're not consuming enough calories: under-eating results in dry hair, dull skin, low mood and poor sleep – hardly a recipe for physical or mental well-being.

It's not easy, with our body-image-obsessed media, but weight mustn't become an overwhelming preoccupation. After suffering from anorexia for a decade, I no longer own a pair of bathroom scales. At long last I've learned to trust myself, to keep a balance, without recourse to that external judgement, those sinister numbers on the dial!

If you listen to your body's appetite and emotions, you'll soon learn what balance feels like. For me, it is a happy place where my body and mind are calm. I'm all too familiar with the warning signs of being too thin; I would start cutting calories and skipping meals, exercising more and sleeping less. Mania would set in, bringing intense bursts of energy, too many ideas, and exhausting highs and lows. My happy, fighting weight is the weight at which my jeans fit, where my periods are regular, and where I can sleep and think clearly rather than being under the illusion of being superwoman.

Eating disorders are increasingly common, and you may be familiar with some of these experiences. Even if you haven't been severely underweight or overweight, you may recognise some of the emotions behind this: judging yourself harshly, allowing your weight to affect your mood. Primal beauty doesn't care if you had a fantastic weekend, indulged a bit and have gained a pound or two. Of course, it's important to maintain a stable weight, but you don't need to weigh yourself every day.

Primal Mantra:
Stop Starving, Start Living

Take a moment to reflect on what beauty means to you. Who is your beauty icon? This could be someone living or dead, of any age: a movie star, a supermodel, singer or an athlete, or just someone you know and love. What is it about them which appeals to you? Is it just their physical appearance, or is there something in their attitude, their personal quirks or style, which makes them awesome? (It's probably nothing to do with their weight.)

And back to the opening question: when have you personally felt at your most beautiful? Try to conjure up a cinematic image in your mind. Focus first on what it was – a specific event, a period in your life – where you were and what you were wearing. Then shift your focus to how you were feeling: what was going on in your life at that time? Where did the beauty come from?

While you're thinking about what makes you feel beautiful inside and out, here's what a few other women said.

> **Marion, 38:** I felt at my most beautiful when I was pregnant with my first child. For the first three months I looked and felt sick as a dog – but when I got past that, and started to look pregnant rather than fat, I felt amazing. Becoming a mother gave me a confidence in my own body I'd always lacked.
>
> **Liz, 27:** I lived in Spain for a few years, first studying and then working. I was in my early 20s and I remember feeling beautiful then. Partly it was the attention from Spanish *señors* – my pale skin and blonde hair seemed to drive them wild! Also, I was eating well, living a healthy outdoors lifestyle, the climate suited me – and I was happy, of course.
>
> **Carla, 47:** I feel beautiful when I've slept. A good night's sleep changes everything – my skin glows, my eyes sparkle, I'm positive and super-productive. It's rare, but when I get a good ten hours I feel like a new person!
>
> Sleep, Spanish sunshine, even pregnancy... There are so many different things that can make women look and feel amazing.

Identify Your Personal Beauty Path

It can be useful to think about your personal beauty secrets – those magic ingredients which you know will make you feel your best. When you're getting ready for a wedding, an interview or a hot date, for example, you probably have routines: whether that's treating yourself to a blow-dry, getting a manicure or maybe buying a new dress.

Then there's everyday beauty: what's your routine between the morning alarm and leaving for work? To put it another way: what could you not face the world without doing? I asked for readers' desert island beauty essentials on Twitter. Here are a few responses:

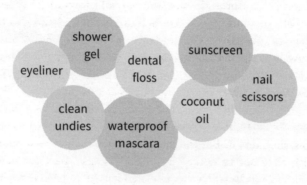

As you can see, everyone has their own preferences and priorities: from eye make-up to fresh pants, we all have different ways of feeling our best. Find a primal beauty routine that works for you, and you'll always start the day on a positive note.

A Question of Cash?

What's your attitude when it comes to premium versus basic beauty? You may find that you're happy with cheaper versions of shower gel or body lotion, for example, but spend more on good-quality facial skincare or cosmetics.

Women's magazines sometimes run questionnaires asking readers about their average annual spend on haircare, cosmetics and tanning, etc. If you've ever added it up, you may have winced at the realisation that you're spending hundreds of pounds a year on the endless matter of hair removal and roots: this is quite literally a never-ending story!

As in many areas of life, beauty is a question of priorities and choice – you might be affluent, comfortable or on a tight budget.

Some people spend their disposable income on a personal trainer or designer gym gear, expensive organic ingredients or eating out at restaurants. Others spend little on their appearance, preferring instead to splash the cash on books, travelling and music or saving for their pension pot.

How Much Is Beauty Worth?

One thing's for sure: despite the global downturn, there's no shortage of premium beauty products, and seemingly no shortage of customers. Many luxury skincare ranges have astronomical price tags and boast some of the rarest ingredients on the planet: anti-ageing creams containing tourmaline and diamond powder, gold, caviar and platinum, with a few tiny vials costing over £1,000.

Most of us wouldn't dream of spending hundreds of pounds, let alone thousands, on face cream. Five or ten pounds should cover most essentials, shouldn't it? But walking around the chemist or supermarket aisles, it's hard not to notice the price difference between male and female beauty products. This female premium hit the headlines in early 2016 – dubbed 'pink pricing', it inflates the cost of everything, from jeans to toiletries to haircuts, simply because they're marketed for the fairer sex – but in reality most women have been aware of it for years.

A great way of going primal is to work out what you need and buy the simplest version – male, female, whatever. Why pay twice the price for pink razors, when the male ones do just as well? The same goes for shampoo and deodorant, if you're not fussy. As if it wasn't bad enough that women are charged more for the basics, we also have to pay for the privilege of menstruating. Why are 'feminine hygiene' products classed as non-essential items, and taxed at five per cent? A baffling list of items which are exempt from UK tax altogether include flapjacks and jaffa cakes, crocodile meat, bingo and houseboat moorings. Even incontinence products, which are arguably closer to sanitary products, attract no tax. (Would things be different if women ran Her Majesty's Revenue and Customs?) Campaigns on social media, such as #BloodyDisgrace on Twitter, have resulted in petitions, websites and a global movement against tampon tax.

There are more primal options: Mooncups are small latex 'cups' which collect the menstrual blood, and can be rinsed and reused. They're far less wasteful, of course, and far better for the environment than traditional sanitary products, but they are yet to become widely popular. While I support everyone's right to choose, and can appreciate how eco-friendly such alternative products are, many of us are glad we don't have to go fully primal with our periods.

Primal beauty is about paring it back, playing up your best bits and not getting the less-than-perfect bits out of proportion. It means keeping things simple. Look at the straightforward routine of your husband, boyfriend, brother or male friends: shower, shave and dress – a squirt of deodorant and maybe a dollop of moisturiser: simple and speedy. Compare that with the plucking and pruning, applying make-up and checking in harsh lights, re-checking from behind, repairing several times a day, the endless hours of drying and straightening hair, the fear of rain and the anxious concealment of fine lines, thread veins or roots. As a friend said the other day, 'Just keeping up with the regrowth and the wrinkles is a full-time job' – let alone striving to look airbrush-perfect.

But primal beauty isn't flawless, and doesn't try to be. These days, consumers are used to seeing airbrushed and retouched images, and we've all been known to use a flattering filter on Instagram. Remember the spate of #nomakeup selfies posted by stunning celebrities who *just happened to wake up like that*?

Whether they were genuinely wearing #nomakeup, the selfies were making a positive point: women don't have to correct, conceal or camouflage their natural looks in order to be considered attractive. After all, if you wear cosmetics or clothes which aren't right for you, you'll feel uncomfortable rather than beautiful.

So what does primal beauty look like? First and foremost, it's entirely self-defined. It's doing what feels right for you, whether that's neatly trimmed and highlighted hair or natural grey streaks, manicure and pedicure, pale and interesting, all-over spray tan, or professionally threaded or waxed. Looks go in and out: perfectly plucked eyebrows have recently given way to much bushier brows; different styles suit different faces and different eras (just look at the perms of the 1980s!). You might change your mind from day to day. I know I do – one day long hair seems sexy and feminine, and the next I want a choppy bob, à la Sienna, Alexa, etc.

You can ditch the rulebook when it comes to primal beauty, because there are no hard-and-fast rules. This is one of the few areas of life where you should feel free to do exactly what *you* want. For example, I hate the caked-on sensation of foundation on my skin, so I use a tinted moisturiser instead. I've never got the hang of lipstick (I look like a clown) but I rely on my black eyeliner and mascara. I prefer cheapo Vaseline to sticky lip gloss, but I pay a lot for my favourite perfume. Maybe you splurge on expensive running shoes, regular haircuts or high-quality vitamins and minerals: it's up to you.

What about getting older? When embracing primal beauty, you can enjoy the life stage you're in, rather than dreading every birthday after the age of 30. It's easy to wax lyrical about the beauty of ageing – female celebrities do it all the time, some through gritted teeth – but actually getting older can be tough. Finding that first grey hair or lion's wrinkle can be hard to 'embrace'. But it *is* a privilege to be alive, after all, and we *can* age with peace and grace. When you stop worrying about age, you can celebrate the milestones of your life – and maybe even laugh at the crow's feet.

> *There will be a day when you look at yourself in a mirror and wonder who that woman is. Surprisingly, you will not tie yourself up in agonised knots about this nor rush out to drop a month's salary on anti-ageing skincare. You might actually celebrate the fact that your skin is the best it has ever been, that your eyes truly are the windows to your soul and that the adorable little scar on your bottom lip, where you pushed your tooth through it at primary school, is not a flaw but part of what makes you who you are.*
> **Helen Walmsley-Johnson, author of *The Invisible Woman***

Glossy magazines have started featuring 'mature' models as the ultimate in edgy chic. The *Guardian* regularly uses 60- and 70-something models in its magazine supplement; even the *Daily Mail* has trumpeted the so-called 'grey emancipation'. On social media, grey hair is popular too, with pictures of silvery locks alongside the hashtag #grannyhair.

Even in Hollywood, the last bastion of sexist ageism, female maturity is becoming less taboo. In the latest Bond film, *Sceptre*, Monica Bellucci plays 007's love interest at <drumroll> the age of 51. An actual Bond woman, not a Bond girl, and near-equal in age to the 47-year-old Bond actor Daniel Craig. Craig himself responded to silly media questions about Bond 'succumbing to the charms of an older woman' by pointing out that they were virtually the same age.

There is still a long way to go: for every successful older actress there are many more who are chucked on the scrap heap after 30. However, these tiny markers of commercial sanity are important. Actresses over 50, including Meryl Streep, Kristin Scott-Thomas and Julianne Moore, are undeniably powerful and increasingly vocal about gender and pay inequality within the industry. It's also encouraging to see fabulous over-80s, including Judi Dench, Maggie Smith and Mary Berry who, at the age of 81, is one of the queens of prime-time television in *The Great British Bake Off*. There is hope for us all!

The Scandinavians are particularly good at mature, natural beauty: my current screen-crush is Trine Dyrholm from the Danish television drama *The Legacy*. Dyrholm plays the delightfully conflicted but stylish character 'Gro'. She has visible lines on her skin – not many, she's only in her 40s – as she has clearly lived a little and laughed; she wears sharp suits and silk dresses, goes after married men, gets hangovers, and generally seems as chaotic as most of us feel whatever our age.

So how do the rest of us feel about ageing beautifully?

> **Libby, 52:** When I turned 50, I just lopped a decade off my age. It wasn't intentional – I was collecting my son from school and one of the other mums said she'd heard I had a big birthday coming

up, and how great I looked for 40. *40?? I was about to turn 50!* I sort of nodded, and ever since then I've thought: why not? You're as old as you feel, right?

Lucy, 35: I don't give a toss about my age. My girlfriend is a few years younger than me but I don't want to be her age, or turn back time, or any of that – every year I live more and learn more – I love the experience and confidence that getting older brings. I'm too busy having adventures to notice wrinkles or grey hairs and that's the way I like it.

Elin, 46: To be frank, I hate ageing. I'm active and healthy, I have an amazing husband and kids, but I still compare myself to other women – friends or just random celebrities in their late 40s and early 50s – and wonder if I look older or younger than they do. I notice the decline in male interest, the occasional flirtatious looks I used to get in cafés or on the street. It makes me feel sad.

Naturally Primal

You probably think a lot about what goes in your mouth, but how often do you stop to consider what goes in your body? The cosmetics, creams and other products you use on your skin eventually find their way into your body, and can affect your health.

The term 'chemical' is something of a misnomer. Commonly used to mean 'bad things we don't want in our bodies', in fact all matter, anything made of atoms – everything inside and outside our bodies – is composed of chemicals. As the website icanhasscience.com explains: 'Anything you can put in a bottle or hold in your hand, anything you can breathe or see or ingest or touch is made of chemicals.' Even water is a chemical.

Pedantry aside, of course we know what we mean when we refer to 'chemicals': those synthetic ingredients, mostly unnecessary and some potentially harmful, which we'd rather avoid. Here are some of the commonest.

Ingredient	Why used?/Why avoid?
Parabens	The most widely used preservatives, you'll see parabens in shampoo, shower gel, body lotion and cosmetics. Parabens are easily absorbed into the skin and can cause allergies and rashes.
Sodium lauryl/ laureth sulfate detergents	Detergents/foaming agents found in shampoo, body wash and toothpaste. Often combined with the chemical TEA , they can cause allergies, skin rashes or irritations. They may be contaminated with the carcinogen 1,4-dioxane.
Synthetic colours and perfume	Often petrochemically based, these are synthetic ingredients used in up to 95 per cent of toiletries and cosmetics. Some colours may be carcinogenic. Perfumes can be neurotoxic and cause headaches, mood swings, depression, dizziness, skin irritation and asthma.
MIT (methyl-isothiazo-linone)	A preservative found in most toiletries and cosmetics. Dermatologists claim it causes severe skin reactions. Also a neurotoxin and potential carcinogen.

Other common ingredients to avoid include: Diazolidinyl urea, imidazolidinyl urea and quaternium-15. They all release formaldehyde and are potentially harmful. If you're concerned about these chemicals, the app Think Dirty has more useful information.

These ingredients make potions and lotions more colourful, fragrant, foamier – and, crucially for the producers and supermarkets, they extend their shelf life. But there are natural alternatives to the harsh colours and preservatives. These products don't just go on and into our bodies, but they're also being washed into the rivers and seas in their millions of gallons. Avoiding the harshest substances is not only good for you; it's also good for the environment.

Do-It-Yourself Beauty

Many of us dabbled in make-your-own beauty experiments when we were children. This usually involved stealing a few avocados from the fridge, mashing them up with honey, spreading the gloopy mixture on your face and waiting for the transformation. Or plundering your mum's best olive oil from the kitchen and mixing it with coarse sea salt, for all-over body exfoliation. The end results of home-beauty efforts were usually pretty messy: I once went to bed with my hair coated in sunflower oil and ruined one of my mum's best pillowcases for evermore.

Not that DIY beauty is any cheaper: a couple of avocados alone cost more than a simple face mask from Boots – and what a waste of those precious fruits! Clearly, we're used to buying ready-made beauty products off the shelf: with busy lives and large families, it's hardly practical to aspire to rustle up bottles of shampoo and body lotion for daily use.

However, just as we make home-made bread or jam for special occasions, there are certain products which are enjoyable to make yourself, such as face masks, and which really reward the effort. Plant oils, essential oils, and floral and herbal extracts are far gentler on the skin and less toxic to the environment. Many of the richest natural ingredients are versatile, widely available and as effective as synthetic alternatives. Here are a few multi-purpose beauty stars.

- **Lavender:** well-known for its calming properties, lavender also stimulates the growth of healthy cells and promotes healing. Lavender floral water regenerates inflamed or damaged skin, and lavender essential oil calms inflammation, dermatitis, eczema and psoriasis. It also reduces stress and anxiety, and encourages restful sleep.

Witch hazel: astringent, cooling and refreshing. It combats excess oiliness, soothes eyes, calms inflamed skin, soothes irritation and roughness, and heals bruises and sores. Rich in antioxidant phenols and tannins.

Rose: ideal for dry, normal and mature skin in a wide range of forms, including rose extract, essentials oils, dried petals and floral water. It supports cell and tissue regeneration, fights bacteria, relieves stress, treats acne and combats signs of ageing.

Honey (also beeswax and other bee products): contains potent healing and antiseptic properties, for use in face masks, skin creams, ointments, salves and emollients.

Tea tree: antiseptic, wound-healing, antibacterial and antifungal. It combats dandruff and body odour, and can be used (diluted) for teeth and gum hygiene and as a mouthwash.

Aloe vera: another cooling and healing remedy – particularly effective for burns and sunburn.

Avocado, coconut and olive oils (and many other oils): rich in healthy fats and nutrients, highly moisturising and healing, they nourish and revitalise the skin. They combat the signs of ageing, condition hair, and repair and protect the skin. These oils are packed with vitamins, minerals, and anti-inflammatory antioxidants. Untreated 100 per cent jojoba oil is excellent for the skin, especially after a day on the beach.

Yarrow: as well as possessing magical properties – on your eyes, it will make you dream of your soulmate; in your bridal bouquet it will grant you a happy marriage – this ancient herb is soothing and cleansing. Use it to remove eye make-up, to ease psoriasis and eczema, to calm rashes and stings, and as an all-purpose balm.

Citrus oils: including orange, lemon, grapefruit and lime. The rinds of citrus fruits are rich in essential oils, which aid detox and weight loss, balance out oily skin and promote a sense of well-being. The zesty aroma of citrus fruits – think bergamot, mandarin, tangerine – are uplifting, invigorating and help to clear the mind.

Water: sounds obvious, but it's vital for glowing skin and hair. Water supports the kidneys to efficiently remove toxins and waste products which cause dull skin. It also hydrates, cleans, tones and improves circulation. Steaming with hot water unblocks pores and clears the airwaves and sinuses.

Also, *be gentle.* Stronger is not always better. Regular exfoliating is all well and good, but you don't need to scrub your body, especially the delicate skin on your face, to shreds. I used a particular brand of toner for years until I talked to a beautician who compared it to paint stripper! It gave me an astringent tingle, but it was far too harsh and stripped away the natural oils. I still like that tingly-fresh feeling of a toner after washing my face, but a simple high-street brand for sensitive skin is fine.

Go Wild for Fruit

Fresh fruit, either eaten whole or used in beauty products, is also full of nourishing natural goodness. Strawberries are full of salicylic acid, vitamin C and AHAs to clear congested skin and balance oiliness. Blueberries are packed with antioxidants. Citrus fruits balance, tone and detoxify, and enhance mental well-being. Olives, pomegranates and apricots are also good for the skin.

Baby Soft

If you don't have the time or the inclination to make your own, baby products are a great alternative. They're formulated for sensitive skin and free of harsh chemicals, containing ingredients such as chamomile, lavender, evening primrose and jojoba oils. Prices range widely, from Boots Baby products to Burt's Bees, Bamford Baby, Lavera and The Organic Pharmacy.

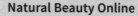

Natural Beauty Online

For more great organic brands (for adults and children) check out:

www.herbfarmacy.co.uk

www.grownalchemist.com

www.fresh.com

www.planetorganic.com

www.naturismo.com

www.beingcontent.com.

Everyday Primal

Primal beauty always starts with the basics: eating well, avoiding stress, and getting adequate rest and good quality sleep. There are also other simple tips for primal beauty.

Less make-up: avoid heavy, clogging foundations and concealers if you can. Mineral make-up is light and gives a natural, even coverage.

Better still, go bare-faced: adapt the 5:2 regime for your skin. Wear make-up no more than five days a week, and aim for two make-up-free days, maybe at weekends. This will allow pores to breathe and skin to rejuvenate.

Daily sun protection: skin needs to absorb vitamin D from daylight, but it also needs good protection against the sun's damaging ultraviolet rays. In extreme temperatures, use a hat and sunglasses, as well as a high-factor sunscreen, and avoid direct exposure.

Drink lots of water: aim for 2 litres (around 3 ½ pints) a day. Tap water is fine, although you may want to use a basic water filter to remove pollutants.

Simple facial massage: ideal for when you're feeling tired and droopy, using some of the essential oils above.

Body brushing: good for sloughing away dull skin cells and encouraging healthy new growth. It also improves circulation, and general skin toning and firming. Before you step in the shower, use a mitt, brush or dry flannel to give your whole body a rhythmic brushing, working upwards, always stroking towards the heart. Massage is also beneficial for your mood and mental well-being.

Good food, including plenty of antioxidants and anti-inflammatory plants: eat flaxseeds, oats and wheat bran to promote clear skin; use nut or rapeseed oils on salads and also in cooking, as a substitute for butter and other vegetables oils.

Go nuts... especially for almonds, Brazil, macadamia and hazelnuts. They're rich in nutrients and healthy fats to keep skin supple and nourished.

When to Splash Out

It makes sense to invest in the products which come into closest contact with delicate areas of skin, and where you need the most care. You might, for example, spend more on a high-quality, high sun protection day cream for your face – and then perhaps compromise on an all-purpose body lotion (especially when your skin is covered up during winter months). As we've seen, the purest organic brands are usually more expensive – like buying organic food, it's a personal choice. (One healthy solution is to use coconut oil everywhere!)

We tend to be suckers for false promises, falling for the idea that something will erase lines, turn back time or reveal our inner goddess. Wherever possible, if something is lush and makes you feel great, make space for it in your life! Add it to your Christmas list (desperate partners will be relieved to know exactly what you want, one-click away on the Internet) or stock up in Duty Free: I buy all my fancy make-up there. Or just treat yourself and use sparingly when you've had a particularly bad day. Unless you're loaded, of course, in which case you can use Crème de la Mer as a hand cream and ignore my thrifty advice.

Healthy Hair

Nutrition matters for your hair just as it matters for the rest of your body. If you're not getting enough high-quality nutrients, that 'crowning glory' will become dull and lifeless, maybe thinning and breaking off, even going prematurely grey. It's no wonder that alternative practitioners look closely at skin and hair as barometers of health or ill-health; our physical well-being reflects the food we eat.

Remember too that hair is fragile – by the time it reaches shoulder-length, it's around three years old. And take a closer look at your habits and products: paraben-clogged shampoos, excessive back-combing or use of extensions, peroxide-based tinting and dyeing products could all be stressing or weakening your hair.

Worst of all are the modern torture implements we inflict on our hair: specifically the blow-drying and straightening tools. As the owner of a pair of ghd straighteners myself, I'm not going to criticise anyone for using them – but the smell of singed follicles should tell you everything you need to know about what they're really doing. In order to make hair poker-straight, these styling tools get to incredibly high temperatures. Have you ever seen women in the 1970s flattening their hair on ironing boards? This is effectively the same thing!

Unlike those irons, the latest hair straighteners now come with protective plates, at least; do use heat-protection products too, when you're styling and straightening. The surest way to avoid hair damage is to stop inflicting heat on it altogether… but at least try not to straighten or blow-dry your hair every day, and always use the coolest setting on your dryer. Whenever possible, leave hair to dry naturally. Embrace the primal look, if you can, and reclaim your right to natural waves, curls or frizz. (Not easy, I know!)

More Primal Pointers for Healthy Hair

Don't wash it every day (or at least take a break at weekends). Over-washing strips natural oils from the scalp, and can lead to thinning, dryness or breakage. Experts say that every other day or every three days is fine (or even less frequently, if you can).

Always rinse thoroughly. When products build up, they can make hair look lank and heavy. After washing, be aware that wet hair is extremely fragile, so comb through gently.

Avoid harsh procedures such as chemical straightening and perming.

Avoid dyeing and stripping products: there are many natural and plant-based alternatives which add glowing tints without damage.

Don't ever bleach your hair (children of the 1990s, our days of Sun-In are behind us!). Use sun protection on the beach, just as you do for your skin.

Always condition: use natural and essential oils, and hair masks, which you can leave in overnight for deep-down conditioning.

Give your hair rest and relaxation: stress boosts androgen hormones which trigger sebum production. Stress can cause hair to fall out, as well as excessive oiliness, dryness, flaky scalp and itching, etc. Sleep is essential for healthy hair.

Massage your scalp: you know when the hairdresser does the 'Indian head massage moment'? Heaven... You can learn your own basic technique, using jojoba or coconut oils, egg yolk, olive oil, yogurt or even honey.

Just as you feed your skin, don't forget to nourish your hair. Eating well strengthens keratin, nourishes the follicles, protects the scalp and brings a shine to your locks. Healthy hair relies on a good supply of protein, iron, zinc, potassium, silica and omega-rich oils. Great food for your diet includes: eggs, oats, spirulina, nettle (in soup/tea), oily fish and nuts. Hazelnuts in particular are a rich source of folate, iron, copper and manganese, vitamin B, biotin, protein and omega-fatty acids. They also contain antioxidant proanthocyanidin for scalp and hair follicles.

Natural Beauty

When it comes to hygiene, you probably want your soap to be 'antibacterial'. But studies have found that the antibacterial ingredient triclosan in many hand soaps can disrupt hormones and the immune system, and may even disrupt fertility. If you're concerned about this, avoid antibacterial sanitiser sprays, gels and soaps. Even if the risks are low, it's not necessary to use such harsh chemicals on your skin. Plain old soap and water are just as effective.

And what about toothpaste? This definitely gets inside your body! Most mainstream brands contain dyes, artificial flavouring, propylene, triclosan and other chemicals. There are natural ranges out there, and they're improving all the time. Be warned: they take some getting used to. I'm currently using an echinacea all-natural toothpaste, and it's a tough switch from the usual stripey minty-fresh taste.

Depending on your level of commitment, you may want to consider using a chemical-free deodorant as well. There have been claims that propylene glycol in mainstream brands, which prevent the product from drying out, are linked to brain, liver and kidney abnormalities. I recently tried a deodorant cream, a blend of vegetable powders, clays, lavender, peppermint and tea tree oil. It smells wonderful and is effective for everyday use, although maybe not for sports or high-stress days...

> **Kath, 42:** I switched because someone told me that regular deodorants are full of anti-freeze... I'd never even thought to look at the ingredients! Now I use a crystal natural deodorant stick. It costs more, but lasts for months. You might need to try a few different brands, and give your body time to adjust. Also it's worth re-applying a few times during the day in hot weather.

Bush Wars

It shouldn't be anyone's business but your own... and yet the discussion over female body hair is more public than ever – specifically in that most private of areas, between your legs. But whether removing body hair is considered a personal choice, a matter of hygiene or a deeply feminist issue, it seems that everyone has an opinion. What is certain is that it can be a time-consuming and expensive process.

The media gets particularly excited about the rights and wrongs of body hair – from Julia Roberts's still infamous red carpet hairy-pits-flash-shocker at a film premiere in 1999 to Instagram's recent decision to ban female body hair. The social media site deleted accounts that showed perfectly innocent photos from women who did not trim their bikini lines – specifically a couple of models whose pubic hair was visible in a swimsuit shot – while taking no action at all on men's pubes or any other male body hair.

Right now it's armpit hair which is making a comeback, with the cool crew not only 'owning' but also flaunting their underarms. Celebrities from Madonna to Miley Cyrus have Instagrammed their unshaven armpits – sometimes even dyeing their underarm hair the colours of the rainbow! It's not only rules over pubes: eyebrows go in and out of fashion too. At school in the 1990s everyone was plucking their brows super-skinny; now it's all about thicker natural brows, à la Cara Delevingne. (Of course, any other facial hair on women remains strictly *verboten*.)

Despite the pressures to conform, some high-profile women are refreshingly relaxed about pubic hair. Gwyneth Paltrow famously claimed to 'rock a 70s vibe' down there, and Cameron Diaz has been honest, even humorous, about why women should keep it natural: 'Pubes keep the goods private, a pretty draping that makes it a little mysterious...' (*The Body Book*).

No woman should feel she *ought* to be hairless – and no man should expect it. Equally, let's not judge women who don't bother, and let's not fetishise underarm hair into a multi-coloured fashion statement.

A straw poll on Twitter reveals a pretty relaxed attitude to body hair from male and female alike.

> **@mr_omneo** I firmly believe women should be comfortable however I'm dismayed at the trend for an aversion to female body hair. #LetItGrow
>
> **@eatingmywayback** nature intended us to have hair where there is hair. It's a misogynist world that makes women feel ashamed of their complete bodies
>
> **@JamesConrad** If you look through the history of Playboy centerfolds, you can see a fullness was the beauty standard up until 1999/2000.
>
> **@DrSamHyde** I think it's up to the individual, but am suspicious of treatments that cause a lot of pain. Torture should not be part of grooming

If we're going truly primal, then you know what I'm going to say about body hair! But that would be hypocritical and inconsistent, because I don't personally rock the cavewoman look. We can't ignore social and cultural norms, and individual preferences: many women prefer to remove a certain amount of body hair, and that's as valid as any other choice. I like smooth legs and underarms, and neatness in the bikini region, but I wouldn't go as far as extreme intimate waxing. I simply don't think it's necessary, and the expectation for adult women to be as hairless as pre-pubescent girls makes me uncomfortable.

From a quick look around the changing room in my local pool, the divide is less exaggerated than the media like to portray. Most of us aren't hirsute cavewomen or porn-star smooth: we all grow hair in the usual places – some more, some less – and most maintain a certain level of 'grooming'. Whether it's a matter of principle or practicality, maybe we don't see the need to be hairless – perhaps we can't stand the pain of waxing, the cost of lasers or the smell of depilatory creams, or we're just too busy to bother.

As my friend Laura says, 'I generally shave my legs in summer, but I don't always bother in winter. And when I have a boyfriend, I'm a lot more lady-scaped than when I'm single.' In other words, it's not really a political or feminist statement: it's about time and hassle, and whether you have bare legs or are wearing thick woolly tights.

It should be entirely your decision, based on what you can be bothered with, what mood you're in and what feels comfortable. No partner, male or female, should ever judge or reject you on something as ultimately superficial as body hair. And if they do – well, you know the answer to that one.

Above All, Enjoy Yourself...

The most important aspect of primal beauty is to remember that you're in control: your appearance is your choice. It's not un-feminist to enjoy make-up and high heels, and neither is it unfeminine to leave your body hair exactly as nature intended. The way you present yourself, the beauty procedures you do (or don't) undergo, the regular upkeep: they are all down to you. Going bare-faced can be as beautiful as wearing make-up; a wild mane of hair can be as stunning as an immaculate sleek bob.

Lots of us enjoy a pampering session in the bathroom, applying our newest skin saviour or illuminating make-up miracle, and that's absolutely fine. There is a legitimate pleasure in taking care of our bodies and experimenting with different beauty treats. Stay positive about ageing and stay primal about products: simple, natural ingredients are good for you and good for the planet. Above all, celebrate yourself: that's the most beautiful look of all.

Chapter 12
Primal Sleep

Q. How many insomniacs does it take to change a lightbulb?
A. None. We just lie in the dark overthinking
every bad decision we've ever made...

Modern life is great for many things, but it's seriously bad for sleep.

If there's one time when we really need to get more primal, it's at night. Look at the way the sun goes down at night and rises in the morning. The nights are longer and darker earlier in winter, when most of us crave more sleep, and shorter and lighter in summer, when we tend to feel more active and energetic.

A 2015 study by Harvard Medical School found that 90 per cent of adults and 75 per cent of children have at least one electronic device in their bedroom. From tablets to laptops to smartphones to let's-just-watch-one-more-episode box sets, the more portable and addictive our devices become, the more they're invading our sleep sanctuaries.

The statistics are startling: according to a report from the World Association of Sleep Medicine, up to 45 per cent of the world's population (or around 3.15 billion people) experience some form of sleep trouble. In the UK, the average person claims to need seven hours and 20 minutes to function at their best, but 70 per cent sleep less than seven hours, and 23 per cent sleep only between four and six hours a night.

Yet sleep is the foundation of our physical, mental and emotional well-being. It's a quiescent period where the body's cells are repairing themselves. Chronic sleep deprivation affects the immune system and hormones, and is linked to colds and flu, diabetes, heart disease, mental illness and even obesity. Not sleeping can impair our mood, outlook and our ability to cope with everyday problems. It affects our everyday lives, from relationships to career prospects to athletic performance, and also our ability to retain information, make decisions, learn and concentrate, our judgement and even our driving technique. Scientists from the University of Surrey compared people who sleep less than six hours a night with those who sleep more than eight and a half, and found that sleeping less altered the expression of 711 genes involved in metabolism, inflammation and immunity and stress. It's even been shown that 20 minutes of sleep deprivation three days in a row can dramatically lower your IQ.

There is virtually no aspect of life that's not improved by better quality of sleep. Hence, the old saying: 'sleep on it' – because almost nothing seems as bad after a good night's rest.

A Modern Obsession

As a society, we're obsessed with sleep. Not only how, when and where other people are doing it, but whether we're 'getting enough'.

Here are a few headlines from recent months.

SLEEP MORE FOR BETTER SEX
longer sleep time linked to greater sexual desire

INSOMNIA MAKES YOU FAT:
sleep loss increases hunger,
affects metabolism and weight loss

**SLEEPING POORLY LINKED TO
ALZHEIMER'S DISEASE AND MEMORY LOSS,**
as brain gets clogged with 'toxic proteins'

6 OUT OF 10 AMERICANS CRAVE SLEEP MORE THAN SEX

TOO MUCH SLEEP COULD LEAD TO AN EARLY GRAVE:
adults who sleep more than nine hours a night
are 30 per cent more likely to die early

NUTRITION AFFECTS SLEEP:
certain nutrients in food affect sleep, from how easy it is
to fall asleep to the quality of rest we get overnight.

Too much sleep can kill – too little sleep can kill – such melodramatic, contradictory messages are enough to keep you awake at night! It's not hard to see why we're confused about sleep. What should be the most natural primal human function has become yet another source of anxiety.

Sleep is for Sissies

We live in an age when lack of sleep has become a weird status symbol. Wall Street mantras like 'you snooze, you lose' have convinced us that busy people don't need cosy naps. Even admitting to being tired can make us feel weak. If you're on the up and up, you don't waste valuable time lying down.

The guilt around sleep has been growing ever since Margaret Thatcher boasted of getting by on three or four hours a night. *Vogue*'s editor Anna Wintour recently let it be known that she's up at 5 a.m. for private tennis coaching and a blow-dry before she starts work. Super-elegant Michelle Obama apparently gets up at 4.30 a.m. for some hard-core cardio. In London, the 'Brutally Early Club' is a select group of movers and shakers who meet at 6.30 a.m. The founder, Hans Ulrich Obrist, describes it as 'a breakfast salon for the 21st century where art meets science meets architecture meets literature'.

The implication is clear: these overachievers are far too important being cultural and cutting-edge pre-dawn to need anything as trivial as shut-eye. So us mere mortals who need at least seven hours (plus the snooze button, a long shower and cereal) are made to feel like we're weak and falling behind. Just like being 'too busy to eat', being 'too busy to sleep' is a sign of power and success. Even the comforting word 'nap' has been hijacked by the super-achievers and twisted into the all-too-brief 'power' nap.

Enough with the competitive not-sleeping! I read a *Paris Review* interview with the Texan writer Mary Karr. Asked about her daily routine, she drawled: 'I nap on a daily basis like a cross-country trucker.' This struck me as admirably honest, hungry, raw. And this is what primal living is all about: grabbing life by the throat, listening to your body's needs and desires, whether it be for food, sleep or sex. In a world of conformity, of being *far too busy* to sleep, Karr's kind of primal honesty is refreshing and healthy. Why do we associate naps with old people? We need sleep to survive so why is it cool to pretend otherwise?

Sleep Trouble

Yet many of us struggle with sleep. It's one of the most instinctive of all human behaviours, but it can be really hard to come by. Unlike walking or talking or eating, reading or writing or riding a bike, we receive no formal instruction on the right or wrong way to fall asleep. Babies are labelled good sleepers or bad sleepers, and then they grow up and are left to get on with it.

Not sleeping can be a desperately lonely experience: it can cause illness, depression, even suicide. Although there is no shortage of well-intentioned advice about hot baths and herbal remedies, many insomniacs find that nothing, except perhaps heavy-duty medication, actually helps. Family doctors can be sympathetic – after all, TATT ('tired all the time') syndrome is one of the commonest reasons for patients to visit their GPs – but again, there is no medical cure for insomnia. Whether a sleep problem is occasional or lifelong, for the sufferer it can feel like being left in the dark.

Worse for Women?

When it comes to sleep trouble, there's a startling gender gap. Despite the fact that women use their brains more during the day, and therefore need more sleep, they're actually getting less. According to Professor Jim Horne, Director of the Sleep Research Centre at Loughborough University, women's busy, multi-tasking brains need around 20 minutes more sleep per night than men.

However, most women aren't getting any extra – quite the opposite. The National Sleep Federation report that 63 per cent of women experience insomnia a few times a week, compared to 54 per cent of men. Also, 58 per cent of women said that pain interrupted their sleep at least three nights per week, compared to 48 per cent of men. Even nocturnal sleep-related eating disorders (midnight sleep snacking) disproportionately affect women, with 66 per cent of sufferers being female.

There are two reasons why women sleep less soundly than men, both of them pretty primal.

1. Hormones: menstruation, pregnancy and the menopause create hormonal fluctuations which can affect sleep.

2. Women also naturally sleep more lightly than men. This may be an evolutionary difference, with females being naturally programmed to wake during the night to feed babies.

Lessons in Sleeping

Last year I attended an insomnia clinic at the Royal London Homeopathic Hospital. This 12-week course (one session a week) is run by one of the UK's leading sleep specialists, Professor Hugh Selsick.

The course started with the basics of 'sleep hygiene': advice about not napping during the day, and tips on lavender pillow spray, warm milk and relaxing baths before bed. We were told that although insomnia is distressing, it wasn't going to kill us. Professor Selsick also reminded us that not sleeping is a common affliction. 'When you're lying awake, you're not alone.' Weirdly, it does help to remember that you're not the only one in your street, neighbourhood or town lying awake. We were asked to keep a sleep log, to draw up graphs of our nocturnal patterns, and to calculate percentages of time spent awake and asleep.

Then came the challenging part: a programme of sleep reduction to improve the efficiency of our sleep. In essence, this involves cutting down the amount of time you spend in bed every night to reduce the amount of time spent lying awake. So, if you're only managing to sleep for three or four hours a night, you gradually shift your bedtime back (e.g. 1 a.m. instead of 11 p.m.) and move your rising time forward (e.g. 5 a.m. instead of 7 a.m.).

This is worse than it sounds. Imagine being forced to stay up until 1 a.m. every night, and then to get out of bed again a few hours later.

You can do anything enjoyable which isn't stimulating or work: reading, painting or listening to music is fine; catching up on emails or paperwork, or watching TV is not. The idea is to avoid lying in bed *awake*, at all costs. As your sleep efficiency improves, you increase the amount of time you spend in bed.

This scientific approach, known as 'sleep restriction therapy' (SRT) is growing in popularity, with some evidence suggesting it's as effective as sleeping pills.

The theory behind SRT makes sense, although I'm not sure how effective it was in practice. Most insomniacs talk of the dread of lying in bed awake, staring into the dark, counting sheep, or counting down the hours until morning, tossing and turning and worrying. The SRT approach breaks that link between wakefulness and bed, making bedtime a less fearful experience. It re-establishes that crucial primal connection between darkness and sleep, preparing us mentally and physically to wind down and power off. I can't pretend that the course changed my life or cured me of all sleeping problems, but it was informative nonetheless. I picked up tips on what to do during those wakeful nocturnal hours, how to worry less about insomnia and some useful relaxation techniques.

The Mystery of Sleep

What is sleep, anyway? The more you think about it, the stranger it seems. It's an altered state of consciousness but markedly different from, say, coma or anaesthesia. Despite the fact that we spend around one third of our lives asleep, neuroscientists admit there is still much we don't understand about the process of falling, and being, asleep – let alone where dreams come from, or what function they serve.

It *is* strange to lie down and sink into unconsciousness on a nightly basis, imagining or recalling vivid events, and then to regain consciousness and go about our daily lives. We're not fully conscious, but we don't completely lose consciousness either. You might assume that the brain switches to standby mode at night, but in fact this isn't the case. In MRI scanners, neurological activity looks quite similar to being awake: our brains are still whirring away, forming images and ideas, conducting conversations, dealing with situations. When sleep experts track the distinct phases of sleep, from the initial lighter sleep to slow-wave sleep (SWS) into the deeper rapid eye movement (REM) and dreaming sleep, the neurons in our brains remain active. Plots in dreams can be as complicated as novels – racy, stimulating or frightening – and yet we accept them as fairly normal and then forget them. In sleep, our olfactory systems are mostly switched off: can you remember tasting or smelling things in dreams?

If you've ever had a general anaesthetic, you'll know that that's different to sleep. When you 'come round' from the operating table, or if you've had concussion or a blackout, you have no idea how much time has elapsed (which is part of the reason it's such a disorienting experience). When waking from sleep, we know that time has passed – we even know roughly how much.

For all that we can't explain about this most essential of human functions, there is plenty we can do to improve it. Taking a primal attitude to your sleep, and making it a priority, is a good place to start.

Circadian Rhythms

Getting back into a more primal relationship with sleep is all about re-establishing those primal circadian rhythms: day, night, light, dark. Here are a few key pointers.

- Maintain a regular sleep-wake cycle. Get up and go to bed at roughly the same time every day, keeping weekdays and weekends consistent.

- Even if you go to bed late, try to get up around the same time each morning – long lie-ins at weekends are tempting, but they can stop you falling asleep at night.

- Similarly, avoid napping during the day if you are prone to insomnia: you want to build up a sleep deficit and get properly tired for bedtime.

- However, stay flexible about your sleep; above all, don't allow it to become an overriding obsession. Don't let it stop you from living your life to the full.

If you're exhausted and have a big night coming up, a cheeky afternoon snooze won't kill you. (I'm a big fan of the disco nap!)

The most important (and hardest) advice to follow is to stop worrying: anxiety increases night-time arousal and traps the brain in self-defeating cycles of worry and stress. Although Professor Selsick reminded us that we wouldn't die from insomnia, many bad sleepers fret all night about everything from world peace to recycling bins to household bills to office troubles to how soon their alarm clock is going off.

Mindfulness for Sleep

Simple mindfulness techniques are shown to reduce anxiety and arousal, and help with falling asleep. These are a combination of breathing and muscle relaxation, as follows.

Detach and relax. When you feel your mind racing, don't try to control your thoughts. Instead, try to detach a little. Distance yourself from your busy brain and don't get caught up: just observe your thoughts and let them go.

Along with this mental detachment, focus on the simple act of breathing. This is an effective technique to distract yourself from over-thinking. Breathe in deeply on a count of three, hold for a short while, and exhale slowly. Count to 20, 50 or 100: you may find you've even drifted off before you reach your target.

Progressive muscle relaxation is another highly effective sleep technique. Starting with your toes, clench each muscle tightly, hold for as long as you can and then release. Feel the difference between tension – when your muscles are clenched – and relaxation. Work your way slowly up the body, through your calves, thighs, buttocks, stomach and all through your upper body. Keep going right up to the muscles in your neck, your jaw and your forehead – we unconsciously hold a lot of tension in our faces.

Progressive muscle relaxation is miraculous: by the end, every part of your body will be thoroughly relaxed, and you'll feel like you're floating. It takes concentration and focus, but is worth the effort. There are many excellent sleep CDs and apps available, some with relaxing music and others which talk you through different visualisation exercises.

Don't Compare

Sleep is very personal; remember that everyone needs different amounts. Most people function best on between six to eight hours of sleep a night, but if you're OK on five hours, or you need nine hours, don't fret. Sleep requirements will vary throughout life as well, depending on your age and activity levels. Newborn babies sleep up to 18 hours a day – albeit in short bursts – because they're going through rapid growth and development. A ten-year-old child needs around 12 hours a night. Adolescents seem to be able to sleep for days on end, new mums are permanently exhausted and sleep-deprived, whereas older people tend to wake early and sleep more lightly.

Above all, try not to measure your nocturnal performance. You wouldn't expect your dreams to be the same as other people's so why compare your sleeping patterns? If you're a light sleeper but you're feeling rested, then you're fine. Of course, you should see your doctor if you're seriously exhausted, depressed or sleepless, as there may be an underlying medical condition.

Stay Calm

Do your best to stay calm even when nothing works. Most of us who battle with sleep find the whole thing intensely stressful. We arm ourselves with the expert advice, get the potions and lotions, drink the right herbal teas and follow the bedtime routines which mostly don't work – and then get even more stressed when we're still awake. Remember that sleep disturbance will probably affect everyone at some stage in their lives, but it's unlikely to last forever.

Try to change your attitude to sleep: for example, *if I drift off, that's great; if not, no big deal.*

As well as progressive muscle relaxation and deep breathing, I sometimes use lying-awake time for productive thinking. I'll start writing an article in my head or plan DIY jobs I need to do, mentally putting up shelves or rearranging furniture. Often when your mind is occupied with mundane thoughts, you drift off naturally.

Keep an open mind. Different things may work for you in different circumstances. When friends or experts recommend books, lavender oils or complementary therapies, don't dismiss them out of hand. Bear in mind that they may feel as frustrated as you, and powerless to help.

Don't let insomnia take over your life. Of course, it's difficult, but it shouldn't stop you from living a full and varied existence. Pledge to do something every day which matters to you – not for your employer or your children, but for you. It doesn't necessarily have to be fun, but it should be something that furthers your personal goals: maybe half an hour learning Spanish on the train, 20 minutes on the exercise bike while watching TV, or writing a few hundred words of that novel. When you're achieving something, you'll be more content and more ready for sleep. Feeling stuck and frustrated is a major source of insomnia. Even if you don't get more sleep, it will feel less important.

Working Out

Physical activity is essential for preparing the mind and body for rest. Exercise triggers the release of chemicals and hormones which improve sleep quality. Late afternoon is an ideal time to exercise, although any time during the day is good. Don't exercise too close to bedtime, as this raises the body's temperature and heart rate, and stimulates adrenalin and brain activity. Above all, stay active – when you're physically tired, you're more likely to drop off.

Food and Drink

Eating well is just as important as exercise when it comes to quality Zzzs. A healthy, balanced diet will give you enough energy to function during the day and switch off at night. Try not to eat just before bed, as this overloads your digestive system at a time when it should be slowing down – but don't go to bed hungry. There's nothing like an empty stomach to keep you awake at night.

Certain foods are known to promote the release of melatonin. You could include them in your evening meal, or as a sleep-inducing bedtime snack.

✓ Turkey and lettuce contain tryptophan, the precursor to melatonin.

✓ Marmite, almonds and oatcakes are also tryptophan-rich, to induce drowsiness.

✓ Honey contains orexin, which reduces alertness.

✓ Bananas also contain high levels of tryptophan, serotonin and magnesium.

✓ Camomile and warm milk are snooze-inducing bedtime drinks.

As well as these sleep-promoting substances, be aware of food and drink which can disrupt sleep. Two important substances to avoid are caffeine and alcohol.

Caffeine is a stimulant found in many foods and drinks – not just coffee – which stays in your system for hours. It's worth bearing in mind that caffeine has a half-life of up to seven hours. This means that if you metabolise caffeine slowly (as many of us do), half the caffeine will still be in your system after seven hours. So that mid-afternoon pick-me-up cup of coffee could well be affecting your sleep. If you're prone to insomnia, limit your caffeine consumption to the morning. If you can't cut coffee out altogether, at least switch to decaffeinated versions after lunchtime. You could see a marked difference in your quality of sleep.

As well as insomnia, caffeine stimulates the adrenal glands and exacerbates stress.

Don't forget that chocolate, tea and many soft drinks also contain caffeine. Green tea is an excellent alternative: it contains around 25 mg of caffeine, compared with 150 mg in a latte. Green tea is also packed full of healthy polyphenols and antioxidants, which strengthen your immune system and protect against cancer and heart disease.

Alcohol is equally troublesome, and not just for the hangover. Although it relaxes you at first, it also dehydrates and disrupts good-quality sleep. Avoid drinking excessive amounts of alcohol, especially right before bed.

Many experts advise keeping a sleep diary, so why not try this for two weeks? It can help you to track the individual factors which may be affecting the quality of your sleep.

A diary is also useful for a doctor or sleep expert to look at your habits and advise on where you might be going wrong.

Fill in your diary every morning, listing events, circumstances and substances that may have affected your sleep. Note down everything: alcohol, caffeine and food consumed, sleeping pills taken, how many trips to the bathroom, and specific anxieties, noise or light disturbance – these are all relevant to your pattern of sleep.

Once you begin to make behavioural or dietary changes, your sleep diary can track improvements. You might notice that you sleep better when you exercise at lunchtime instead of the evening, for example, or when you cut out coffee in the afternoon.

Alternative Remedies

Alternative therapies may relieve insomnia. Although the evidence is more anecdotal than scientific, it's worth a try. Acupuncture, massage, reflexology and homeopathic remedies often promote relaxation, which in turns aids sleep. Valerian, taken at night as herbal sleeping pills or as a drink, is also thought to be effective.

Cave-bedroom

Think primal when it comes to your bedroom: the more cave-like, the better. I don't mean to suggest that you should actually sleep on hard rocks under animal skins, but it should be cool, well-ventilated and dark. If possible, invest in the best bed linen. It's hardly cave-like, but the more comfortable you feel at night, the better you'll sleep. You spend around a third of your life in bed, so don't economise on a mattress or pillows. Buy a range of lighter and warmer sheets and duvets for different seasons.

If you're sharing a bed, consider buying a mattress with 'split' sections to reduce 'motion transfer'. We all toss and turn during the night, and it's no good bouncing around every time your bedfellow moves. Go for innerspring, memory foam, extra-firm or super-soft – whatever works for you.

The emphasis should be on quiet, calm and comfort. It can help to think of your bedroom as a sleep-cave, a place to retreat from the outside world. This cave is a sanctuary for sleep and sex, resting and dreaming. This image will help to reinforce your most primal sleep instincts, inducing a sense of natural drowsiness as night falls. It will also encourage your body to produce the sleep hormone, melatonin, which promotes restful sleep. Lastly, it will help to reset that body clock: re-establishing the day/night and light/dark cycles which modern life can interrupt. As we'll see, these cycles are essential to our primal circadian rhythm.

Respect Your Rhythms

There is much scientific evidence on the damaging effects of technology on our sleep patterns. Sleep cycles are regulated by circadian rhythms, which are in turn regulated by light and darkness. Melatonin is a hormone produced by the pineal gland in the brain and it plays a key role in making us feel sleepy. Tablets, smartphones, laptops and televisions emit blue light: a short-wavelength light that has been found to interfere with the production of melatonin. Staring at a bright screen for two hours makes the body release 22 per cent less of this essential sleep hormone.

Electronic devices in the bedroom give our bodies and brains confusing signals, blocking the natural production of melatonin and thus interfering with our natural sleep cycles. We are artificially wakeful but simultaneously sleep-starved. No wonder many of us are left feeling exhausted but unable to power down.

You know this, but it bears repeating anyway: ban electronic devices from your bedroom. You shouldn't be watching TV in there and certainly not taking your laptop or smartphone to bed. Charge your gadgets in another room. Avoid the evil, energising blue lights which disrupt melatonin and fool your body into thinking you need to stay awake. Strictly speaking, you shouldn't even listen to the radio (although for many insomniacs this can be a hard habit to break).

Think primal: there is no daylight at this time, so avoid switching on artificial lights or watching flashing/stimulating films. Use nightlights or dim lighting in the bedroom (I use candles) and, if possible, avoid switching on the overhead bathroom lights in the middle of the night. When you wake in the morning, open the curtains and windows to let natural light pour in, to reinforce your body's natural circadian rhythms.

> **Dr Tim Quinnell, Consultant at Papworth Hospital's Sleep Centre:** 'Wind down properly. If you can't sleep because your brain is whizzing, make an effort to disengage from the outside world an hour or two before bedtime. Stop working, come off social media, stop surfing the net, and try more relaxing activities such as chatting or having a bath. You could do a "mental download" – write down everything that is whirring around in your head, to help your brain go into neutral.'

> Sleep Cycle tracks your sleep patterns throughout the night to determine the best time to wake you up. Based on research into the 90-minute sleep cycles – light sleep, deep sleep, REM/dreaming sleep – the app will wake you when you're in the lightest stage of sleep. This makes you feel like you woke naturally without an alarm clock (you set a 30-minute window of when you need to get up) so you feel more refreshed and less jolted awake. The app also creates charts of your sleeping patterns to identify any problems.

Primal Morning Routines

On the subject of sleep and waking, celebrity explorer Bear Grylls, Mr Primal himself, dislikes the label *alarm clock*: 'Alarm to me says "emergency" and that my life is in danger. That's a terrible way to start the day! I call it, instead, my "opportunity" clock. Waking me up to give me the opportunity to get out there and grab life with both hands.'

You might not embrace mornings as fully as Bear Grylls, but he raises an interesting idea. Mornings are a great opportunity for calm, grounding and reflection. Hopefully, once you're sleeping more primally, you'll feel more energetic when you wake. Just as primal night-time routines can improve the quality of your sleep, so positive morning routines can set you up for the day.

Here are a few simple habits which will transform your day. Try to do them every morning before 9 a.m. They will make you feel healthier, happier and less hectic.

1. **Get an early start:** if you find you're always rushing in the morning, make an effort to get up slightly before the usual time. Go to bed earlier and set your alarm for half an hour – even ten minutes – earlier in the morning. Don't fill this extra time with more chores: just savour the quiet with no interruptions or commitments.

2. **Meditate and give thanks:** begin each day with love, grace and gratitude. You can write down your thoughts (morning pages) or simply sit in silence and think about the blessings in your life. The habit of thankfulness is addictive: soon you'll start to see good things all around you all day long. Remember: 'It's not happiness that makes us grateful, but gratefulness that makes us happy'.

3. **Stretch and breathe:** you may like to exercise in the early morning – I love to swim first thing – or simply have a good, long stretch. Inhale and exhale, feel the pulling sensation in every limb. You could incorporate a few basic yoga moves: sun salutations and downward dog are perfect early-morning moves. Stretching will increase your flexibility, energy, muscle co-ordination, concentration and all-round well-being.

4. **Drink water.** Before you consume anything else, drink a large glass of water! Our bodies are made up of 60–70 per cent water, so it's important to rehydrate after a night's sleep. You may prefer hot water with a slice of lemon, or cold water (not iced) – but make sure that you drink it before tea, coffee or breakfast.

5. **Avoid technology, newspapers, radio and TV.** Keep your phone switched off, don't go on social media (especially not to Instagram your awesome morning stretching!) and don't check voicemail or emails. This is tough for those of us addicted to a morning dose of news and politics, but give yourself at least 15 minutes of peace and quiet.

6. **Above all, keep it simple:** don't overschedule your early mornings. The whole point about this extra time is that you're *not* trying to juggle a million tasks (as many of us do during the working day). Don't try to accomplish too much: remember that this is your space to think and feel; just write a few lines, read something inspiring, stretch, breathe, drink your water and savour the silence.

The Benefits of Primal Sleep

If there's one area of life where your simple adjustments will reap immediate results, it's in your sleep. By adopting a few primal habits, you can change your daily sleeping – and waking – experience from a weary struggle to a positive pleasure. A few nocturnal tweaks could help you to sleep like a log and rise with a spring in your step.

We're all guilty of allowing the anxieties and distractions of the outside world to creep into our homes, by bringing work back from the office, staying up late staring at digital devices or binge-watching box sets. All of these habits can make us feel more wired and wakeful. While we can't avoid the external stressors and recreations of modern life altogether, we can keep one room as a sanctuary: disconnected, dark and indulgently comfortable.

The benefits of primal sleep go far beyond those hours of darkness: when you sleep better, you eat better, and have more energy for work, exercise and relationships. Quality sleep improves your mood, concentration and cognitive performance – and is a natural beauty booster too, giving you glowing skin and sparkling eyes. Redesigning your bedroom into a true temple of sleep can be transformative for every aspect of your mental and physical health.

Next time you find yourself texting, tweeting or emailing from your bed late at night, with the TV or radio blaring and artificial lights on, stop and ask yourself whether this is really the time and the place… Remember: this isn't your living room, office or media centre: this is your sleep-cave. It's not that hard to leave mobiles and laptops in another room. Take yourself back thousands of years: what would cavemen do?

Chapter 13
Primal World

In June 2015, Pope Francis hit the headlines with a radical encyclical about the global environmental crisis. In it he lyrically described 'the cry of the earth, the cry of the poor'.

It was the first time any global religious figure had issued such a comprehensive statement: in no uncertain terms, the Pope blamed the crisis on collective human selfishness, recklessness and, above all, the indifference of the powerful.

The Pope highlighted the fact that although climate change is created by the wealthy, it disproportionately affects the world's three billion poorest people. 'Those who possess more resources and economic or political power seem mostly to be concerned with masking the problems or concealing their symptoms.'

The Pope's climate change encyclical clearly touched a nerve, not only among his Catholic flock, but also among other Christians, Muslims, Jews and those without any religious beliefs. It called for every one of us to play our part in conserving the world in which we live, and in healing some of the damage we have already done.

Despite the challenges ahead, we can all take positive, primal action. The Pope's statement made such an impact – even trending on social media – because he spoke to us on a human, individual level. It reminded us that our choices really matter, not only to the planet, but also to our fellow human beings.

It may be uncomfortable to acknowledge that what we do has an impact on the environment – whether that's driving, flying, eating meat or having a lot of children – but living in a more primal way means asking ourselves some hard questions, such as the following.

When I use all those plastic bags to carry my stuff back from the supermarket and throw them away, where do they end up?

When I fill up my car, where does the petrol come from? Also, what comes out of the exhaust pipe, and where does it go to?

When I casually have bacon for breakfast, a ham sandwich for lunch and a chicken salad for dinner, where does all that meat come from?

The answers to questions like these are far from straightforward. But even asking them is an important first step in developing a more primal attitude to our planet. What difference can we actually make?

Climate change sceptics argue that our efforts are futile. They insist that, however we act at a local level, the majority of oil consumption and carbon emission occurs in the United States and in developing countries such as China and India, as their industries grow, populations increase and living standards improve. The sceptics declare that installing solar panels on every roof in Europe wouldn't make much difference. Your tiny efforts to go green, your insignificant non-polluting little bike rides are pointless – a drop in the ocean of the global warming problem.

Again, this is where the primal attitude comes in. We all have a responsibility to keep this Earth in good shape – and we *can* all make a difference. If everyone does nothing, nothing changes; if we all do a little, we can change a lot. The environment is one of the most intractable issues of our age; for non-scientists it can be hard to work out what's really going on. Finding solutions to these knotty problems is not going to be simple.

However, it is not beyond us: scientists, philosophers and governments can achieve incredible things when they want to. Neither is money the issue here: we spend billions of dollars on space exploration, and billions more on drones, bombs and nuclear weapons. Sure, the findings from Pluto are exciting, and yes it's thrilling to imagine humans one day travelling en masse to the Moon... But how about we deal with the problems we've created on our own planet before we go exploring others?

Just as a journey of a thousand miles starts with a single step, so every one of us can make a positive difference. Let's start by looking at how we're living now and what practical changes we can make.

From extreme weather to air pollution, polar bears to papal proclamations, concern over climate change is at an all-time high. According to the World Wildlife Fund, since 1970 populations of mammals, birds, reptiles, amphibians and fish around the globe have dropped 52 per cent. The *Financial Times* recently reported that China will need to spend $1.1 trillion to clean up its contaminated soil; it is literally becoming too polluted to feed itself. (It should be noted that although China is the world's biggest carbon polluter, it's also the world's leading investor in wind, solar and other renewable energies. In 2015 a report from the London School of Economics suggested that China's greenhouse gas emissions may start to fall within the next decade, five years ahead of target.)

This is no longer a future crisis, to be dealt with next century, next decade or at the next global summit: in many parts of the world, catastrophic climate change is happening *right now*. The ecological footprint per person, in high-income countries, outweighs the planet's biocapacity to cope. In 2015 Delhi endured weeks of punishing heatwave, with temperatures over 45°C, before Chennai experienced their worst floods in half a century. The future of the Arctic, one of the few remaining pristine corners of the Earth, hangs in the balance too. Shell recently shelved plans to start drilling for oil there... for now.

Whether it's extreme heat in India, droughts from California to North Korea, species extinction or fracking beneath the British countryside, all of us are affected. This is no longer just a scientific theory but a daily reality: in 2015, scientists chillingly announced 'the sixth mass extinction has begun'. UK meteorologists recorded the hottest ever July day (36.7°C) and made this alarming prediction: by the end of the twenty-first century, the probability of these very hot summers occurring will rise from 25 per cent to around 90 per cent. Globally, 2015 was the warmest year on record. The UK Met Office estimates 2016 will be at least as hot as 2015, which would signal the three hottest years ever recorded in a row.

It's estimated that between 95–97 per cent of scientists now agree that global warming is real, and man-made. Witness the gradually submerging islands in the Maldives, rising sea levels, melting polar ice and extreme weather events. Some sceptics still disagree, arguing that the Earth's temperature fluctuates naturally, and always has done, through warmer and cooler (and icy) ages, and that recent rises of a few degrees are no more than a blip. While they're correct in saying that temperatures have always varied slightly, the overwhelming consensus is that we're now seeing something more significant than the natural fluctuations of previous centuries.

We're certainly experiencing more extreme weather at both ends of the spectrum – from floods to typhoons to droughts – and there is no longer much doubt that the ongoing uses and abuses of our natural environment are having dire consequences. The evidence of pollution is all around us, in our seas, skies and on our streets. Clearly, the time for action is overdue. We cannot go on destroying fragile species and their habitats, polluting air, land and oceans, producing greenhouse gases and causing climate change, and losing forest, prairies, savannahs and wetlands.

The question is more urgent than ever: what kind of Earth are we leaving for future generations?

The Way We Live Now

Whatever else we do, we need to start looking at the direction in which we're heading. In the developed West, we consume and discard at an alarming rate. Plastic was only invented in the 1950s but in the last 60 years we've converted to a grab'n'go society, hooked on the stuff: every sandwich we buy and practically every carrot, potato or apple comes nestled in unnecessary layers of cellophane packaging, to say nothing of the endless plastic bottles. Overall plastic production reached 311 million tonnes in 2014.

The amount of litter in the oceans is truly shocking. In January 2016 the Ellen MacArthur Foundation reported that one refuse truck's-worth of plastic is dumped into the sea every minute and that by 2050 there will be more plastic in the world's oceans than fish, by weight. Even in the remotest waters, in the most far-flung corners of the Earth, you'll find a fine layer of debris floating just below the surface – scraps of plastic, bits of cellophane, water bottles, wisps of balloons and rubber gloves. You see this kind of trash strewn everywhere from the English countryside to the Egyptian desert. Plastic has transformed manufacturing, medicine and everyday lives, but it's also one of the scourges of the modern world.

> ❝ Plastic bags can take years to fully decompose and even though household recycling rates have improved significantly in recent years, 16,000 tonnes of waste still goes to landfill every year. Around eight million tonnes of plastic also ends up in our oceans each year, polluting our marine environment and harming our precious sealife. ❞
> **Department for Environment, Food and Rural Affairs**

Plastic can damage human health, as well as the environment. Recent scientific research has uncovered alarming links between common chemicals found in sunscreen and clothing, and male infertility. In June 2015 Niels Jørgensen, consultant at Rigshospitalet, Copenhagen, said that we should be 'very worried' about declining sperm quality in men across Europe. Tests showed that chemicals such as phthalates and PFCs – found in plastics, shower curtains, raincoats, suncream, car dashboards and cleaning materials – have an effect on semen quality. Studies in Denmark suggest that sperm counts are 25 per cent lower than in the 1940s because of the widespread use of chemicals, and a 1992 study showed a 50 per cent decline in sperm quality over the last 50 years. At a primal level, the chemicals in our environment are affecting the very building blocks of new life.

How did we get so hooked on plastic? One of the biggest uses, of course, is plastic carrier bags. Across most of Europe it's completely normal to take cloth bags to the supermarket. My brother, who lives in Frankfurt, says: 'I'd be astonished if my wife or kids came home carrying plastic shopping bags. It might have been an inconvenience at the very start, but these days it's just a habit – the same way you grab your wallet and car keys, you grab a couple of cloth bags.' Living more primally – recycling and reusing bags, for example – is easy once you get into the habit.

In recent years, the plastic bag problem has been reaching epidemic proportions. In July 2015 the *Daily Mail* reported: 'the number of "plastic poison" carrier bags given away by supermarkets soared by 200 million to 8.5 billion... supermarkets are giving out an average of 11 bags for every person in England every month... the average household already has 40 plastic bags stashed away in cupboards.'

We've all seen images of seabirds entangled or choking on plastic bags, or drowning in spilled oil. Around the world, an estimated one million birds and 100,000 marine mammals and sea turtles die each year when they become trapped in plastic or eat it. There are believed to be 13,000 pieces of plastic litter per square kilometre of the world's oceans: and it kills marine wildlife. In 2012, a young sperm whale was found dead, floating off the coast of Greece. It was discovered that his stomach was full of 100 plastic bags.

Organisations like WRAP, Ban the Bag and the Marine Conservation Society have long campaigned for retailers to charge for plastic bags. Finally, in October 2015, a 5p levy on plastic bags was introduced in the UK (following Scotland and Northern Ireland's example). The results have been outstanding: by the end of 2015, the British Retail Consortium reported that plastic bag usage among the major supermarkets had dropped by more than 75 per cent. It's also an encouraging example of how determined environmental campaigning has brought about significant change. Something as simple as a 5p charge made us realise that we didn't really need those plastic bags after all – reusable ones would do just fine.

To Frack or Not To Frack?

Plastic is made from polymers, most of which are derived from oil and gas. How much of the planet's natural resources have we used up, and how much remains? What happens when we've used up all the oil, coal and gas?

No one can predict the precise date of 'peak oil' – the point at which we reach maximum oil production before reserves begin to enter an irreversible decline – but there is no doubt that we're consuming fossil fuels at a frightening rate. Global daily oil consumption increased from 63 million barrels in 1980 to 85 million barrels in 2006. Industry experts argue that now we've accessed most of the 'easy' and 'cheap' oil and gas reserves, and we need to start looking at more ingenious ways to get at the rest.

Hence the new (and highly controversial) technique of fracking, which involves drilling into the Earth, before directing high-pressure water at the rock to release gas from inside. The *Guardian* journalist Ian Martin described frackers as: 'The ones who drill deep beneath that area of local countryside... who then pump into the ground powerful jets of high-pressure hydrogunk, splintering rock as easily as a walnut. And who, having sucked up a sky's worth of valuable gas through a massive crack pipe, then pack up and lumber off to fracture and steal someone else's treasure.'(The *Guardian*, 30 June 2015)

Anti-fracking groups across the UK and US raise serious concerns about this practice, and have even linked it to earthquakes (although the evidence is not conclusive). The current UK government is 'committed' to the pursuit of shale gas, much to the dismay of Greenpeace and other environmental pressure groups. In late 2015 the government granted 159 licences for onshore oil and gas exploration, many in the north of England (although there is a moratorium against fracking in Scotland). Ministers also gave the go-ahead for fracking under many of our National Parks. Greenpeace responded by saying: 'The UK government's gung ho approach to a new fossil fuel industry is bizarre and irresponsible... And now that fracking under National Parks and other protected areas has been pushed through – it seems that nowhere is sacred.'

The arguments are divisive: it's simplistic to portray the frackers as capitalist monsters and anti-frackers as tree-hugging hippies. As consumers, we have to take responsibility, since we all rely (for now) on oil and gas. But we cannot ignore the facts that fracking has been linked (although not conclusively) to several recent earthquakes across the United States. For many of us, there is something alarming about the prospect of high-pressure drilling, splintering and fracturing, thousands of feet beneath our rural landscapes and National Parks. In a primal sense, shouldn't we be trying to keep our planet in one piece?

Polluted Planet

According to George Monbiot, climate change is the 'moral question of the 21st century'. The British environmental activist and writer has spent decades calling for the reduction of greenhouse gas emissions, the construction of offshore wind farms, more efficient public transport systems and an end to all new road-building.

Think this sounds extreme? Monbiot also wants to ban patio heaters and garden floodlights, issue every citizen with a 'personal carbon ration', close down all out-of-town superstores, and reduce UK airport capacity by 90 per cent.

Your reaction to his ideas will probably be instinctive and immediate. You may roll your eyes and think he's barmy and unrealistic. Or you may (like me) think *YES! Let's do it...*

Be the Change

It is hard for us as individuals to influence international or even national policy on such global problems as pollution and carbon emissions. However, we're not powerless. There are numerous easy wins in the environmental battle: changes which you can make immediately, and which will make a difference. Monbiot singles out wasteful luxuries, such as patio heaters, and the same goes for washer-dryers. It is simple to string up a washing line in your garden or balcony, or even across the bathroom. In winter, you can use clothes racks and airing cupboards. That's a really simple primal change you can make to reduce energy consumption right now.

There are easy energy savings to be made on a larger scale, too: look at the night skyline of any big city and you'll see thousands of empty office buildings, brightly lit and needlessly burning electricity. While safety lights are needed at night for aircraft, multi-storey skyscrapers do *not* need to be fully illuminated. The same goes for excessive air conditioning: in Hong Kong some buildings are so fiercely air-conditioned that cinemas actually hand out blankets. The scandal of this kind of energy consumption is that it's manifestly unnecessary. If we care about preserving our planet, we must challenge this squandering of precious primal resources. From individuals to corporations, every choice matters.

Three Trillion and Falling

Or what about planting a tree? It's estimated that there are currently three trillion trees on Earth, eight times more than the previous best guess (Yale University, September 2015). This is around 422 trees for every human being. However, scientists also found that tree cover has nearly halved since the start of human civilisation. The pace of deforestation has not decreased: our species is currently felling around 15 billion trees every year.

It's been shown that simply looking at trees helps the body to recover faster, reduces stress, balances hormone production and slows heart rate. Nature is a powerful healer: studies have shown that greenery in the environment brings wealth, as well as health, benefits. Researchers in Toronto found that people living on tree-lined streets reported health benefits equivalent to being seven years younger or receiving a $10,000 pay rise, and US scientists have linked trees to improvements in mental health and asthma.

In short, trees really matter: for humans, for the planet and for the economy. They raise house prices, look pretty, store carbon, remove carbon, hold rainwater and even balance extreme temperatures. How many more reasons do we need to make our towns and cities greener?

Global Action?

I was in Copenhagen for the 2009 Climate Change Conference, and I remember the disappointment over the international failure to take any meaningful action. However, progress has been made since then. At the G7 meeting in Bavaria in June 2015, the world's seven richest nations predicted the death knell for fossil fuels by the end of the twenty-first century. They set out a vision of the total decarbonisation of the global economy, with emissions being cut in half by 2050, and completely by 2100. As with previous positive developments, however, this agreement was non-binding and unfeasibly long-term (after all, which government is going to be around to account for their actions in 2100?). Environmental activists and scientists called these vague commitments 'recklessly complacent'.

There was a ray of hope from one of the Earth's big polluting countries in late 2015. Launching his 'clean power plan', President Obama said: 'There is such a thing as being too late when it comes to climate change', arguing that we may be the last generation who can actually do anything to tackle this global threat.

Whatever its shortcomings, the Paris Climate Change Conference was seen as crucial. Two weeks of intensive negotiation between 195 nations resulted in what world leaders called 'the single most important collective action for addressing climate change ever agreed upon'. Here are the key outcomes:

- to ensure that global warming stays 'well below' 2°C and to 'pursue efforts' to limit the temperature rise to 1.5°C

- by some point after 2050, to reduce man-made emissions to a level that forests and oceans can absorb

- to agree to set national targets for reducing greenhouse gas emissions every five years

- all countries – both developed and developing – to report on their efforts to reduce emissions; no penalties for countries that miss their emissions targets, but 'transparency rules' to encourage progress

- wealthy countries to continue to offer financial support to help poorer countries reduce emissions and adapt to climate change; emerging economies, such as China, to contribute on a voluntary basis (however, no specific dollar amounts set)

a recognition of 'loss and damage' suffered by small island nations from climate-related disasters; however, 'loss and damage' would not involve liability or compensation.

So, is this enough to save the planet or just a disappointing compromise? It's hardly the radical action Pope Francis and many others had called for, but it does represent gradual progress on the part of governments around the world, both in facing up to the scale of the environmental crisis and to begin taking action.

Boycotting Plastic

The more plastic we use, the more we must produce: most of it is entirely unnecessary. Just as being more primal encourages you to consume the freshest produce you can, so it asks you to think more critically about the composition of every product you buy. Taking a primal attitude to the environment means noticing your casual daily plastic consumption. The phrase 'boycotting plastic' sounds rather militant, but cutting down radically on the packaging you allow into your life is entirely within your control, and it feels wonderfully primal.

Here are a few other ways in which you can cut your consumption of plastic (or at least mitigate the damage).

✓ Leave your fruit and vegetables loose where possible – try to use fewer individual plastic bags.

✓ Take re-usable bags every time you shop: it's easy to leave a couple of cloth bags in the boot of your car or under your desk.

✓ Avoid buying small bottles of water, or refill them when you do (the UK's tap water is safe!).

✓ Recycle plastic waste properly – and don't ever release balloons or Chinese lanterns into the sky (they have to fall to earth/sea).

✓ Sign petitions to reduce the widespread use of plastic packaging (you can find these on the websites of Greenpeace, Rainforest Rescue and many others).

Living in a primal way means thinking seriously about how we can use fewer of the Earth's precious resources. It's not just about our fossil fuel consumption: living primally means not polluting our oceans and our skies, and not filling the Earth with landfill, covering it over and forgetting about it. It means not buying and discarding, not consuming endlessly, not acting as though we're the only ones who matter. It means not wasting food: not expecting to eat meat every day, not throwing away fruit and vegetables, and being creative with cooking and freezing food.

It means thinking about the generations who will follow us, and how they will live, eat and work. It means caring about our local environment too: local parks, green spaces, urban places. It means travelling in greener ways if possible – using bikes and public transport instead of cars – and yes, maybe it means flying less often or offsetting carbon emissions where possible. It means caring about our environment, and composting, recycling and reusing.

Of course, we all lead busy lives, but simple changes make a significant difference. Living more primally, with a lighter footprint, doesn't have to be time-consuming. It doesn't have to be expensive either – in fact, cutting your energy consumption will reduce your household bills. Make it a priority, and soon it will become second nature.

Elixir of Life

Oil may be profitable, but water is the source of all life on Earth. And yet, with our access to apparently unlimited running hot and cold water at the turn of a tap, it's too easy to waste. The average household uses around 130,000 gallons of water per year – the average individual around 70 gallons per day – and things are getting worse. In 1990, 30 states in the US reported 'water-stress' conditions. In 2000, this had risen to 40 states, and by 2009, it was 45 states. Some states are literally running out of water: California has been experiencing severe drought since 2013; in January 2015 Governor Jerry Brown declared a drought state of emergency and imposed strict conservation measures. On the other side of the world, North Korea is experiencing severe drought conditions and widespread crop failures.

Our access to water may feel 'unlimited' but of course it's not. If only we could treat water as our primal ancestors did, as something we had to source and even carry ourselves. I love water – from morning swims to relaxing bedtime baths – and nothing makes me happier than the view of an ocean, a lake, river or canal. If I could live by the sea, I would. But sometimes it's easy to forget what a precious resource it really is. If there is one straightforward, non-technical, free place to start with living primally, it's ending water wastage.

There are numerous ways to use and reuse water. We mainly use water in the bathroom: this accounts for around 75 per cent of household water usage. Around 25 per cent goes down the toilet, as we flush away 2 billion litres of water per day in the UK. And down the plughole: in the 1970s less than 20 per cent of UK homes had a shower, whereas today that number has risen to 85 per cent.

There are plenty of water-saving gadgets available online, such as 'low flow' shower heads, dual flush toilet attachments and aerators for kitchen taps. A friend gave me a nifty device, a five-minute 'sand timer', which you attach to the bathroom tiles with suckers, like an hourglass. You flip it over and when all the sand has run through, that's your shower done. The average person's shower time is eight minutes, so this helps to reduce energy and water usage, and trying to beat the clock is fun (children especially love it!).

Other Tips for Conserving H_2O

✓ Switch off the tap when brushing your teeth: a running tap wastes over 6 litres of water per minute.

✓ Use cold water instead of hot water where possible.

✓ Replace deep baths with quick showers.

✓ When washing up by hand, don't leave the hot tap running continuously: fill the sink instead.

✓ Fix leaky washers: a dripping tap wastes around 5,500 litres of water a year.

✓ Only run the dishwasher and/or washing machine when you have a full load.

✓ Always use the 'eco' settings on washing machines and dishwashers.

✓ And remember: UK tap water is *safe to drink*. Use filter jugs if you prefer, but don't buy bottled water. In hot weather, fill bottles of drinking water and store them in the fridge.

... And in the Garden

✓ Sprinklers can use up to 1,000 litres of water per hour. If necessary, use them early morning/late afternoon, when evaporation rates are lowest, and don't water when windy.

✓ Install a water butt (or an upturned barrel) in your garden or on your balcony: this collects precious rainwater which you can use to water the plants.

✓ Reuse bathwater or kitchen water on the garden (but not on fruit or vegetables).

✓ Use mulch and bark in your garden: this can reduce evaporation by up to 75 per cent.

✓ Lawns can and should be allowed to go brown occasionally: it helps to build up resistance and recover immediately after rainfall.

These are small, manageable adjustments that we can all make at home and which, collectively, will save millions of gallons of water every year. Not only will they save us money on utility bills, but they also help to mitigate the ongoing pollution of lakes, rivers and reservoirs. The more water we use, the more dirt, detergent, medication, hormones and human waste find their way into the environment. The less we use, the better.

Quick and Easy Eco-tips

✓ Turn down the heat: lowering your thermostat by a few degrees has a real impact on overall fuel consumption. Good for the planet, good for your bills and good for your body, too.

✓ Bye-bye standby: don't leave your electronic gadgets plugged in overnight. Unplug them when they're fully charged (for phones) and switch them off at the socket when they're not in use (for TVs, DVDs, etc.). As above, this will save you money, as well as energy.

✓ If you can cycle or walk to the shops, to the office, to university or to your children's school, DO! It's reliable, invigorating – and free. You can count it as part of your daily exercise and feel virtuous in the knowledge that no fossil fuels were burned during your journey. Cycling and walking will give you toned muscles, as well as a bloom in your cheeks.

✓ Keep your phone on eco/battery-saving mode.

✓ Use refills: buying coffee refills instead of glass jars saves 97 per cent of packaging waste.

✓ If you shop at wholefood markets or greengrocers, many will be happy to let you refill your own containers. This works perfectly for cereals, lentils, rice, seeds, herbs and spices.

✓ Avoid cheap/fast fashion stores which sell jumpers, dresses and T-shirts for as little as a few pounds. Most of these disposable garments are poor quality, and not worth re-selling, so they end up in landfill. Many are also produced using exploitative labour.

✓ Second-hand/vintage shops are a great way to assuage your retail guilt; try to operate a one-in, one-out policy, and when you're buying, you know you're contributing to charity and reusing.

Be Greener and Leaner

Rethink your plate: make vegetables and/or salad a more prominent part of every meal. Experimenting with seasonings and salad dressings can make this healthiest produce taste amazing.

Grow your own: whether you have a garden, a balcony or just a windowsill, you can cultivate a surprisingly wide range of vegetables or herbs. If you're really pressed for outside space – and many city-dwellers are – then have a look at some easy-to-grow vegetables listed below. With a little ingenuity and organisation, you could soon find yourself becoming self-sufficient. Nothing tastes as good as something you've grown yourself. If you really have no space at all, you can even sow watercress on a damp flannel – bring on the delicious egg and cress sandwiches!

Herbs: simple to grow, and they smell and taste wonderful. Start with oregano, basil, mint, thyme and rosemary, and use them instead of salt. Plant them in a window box for accessibility and fragrance – it's a joy to be able to open your kitchen window and snip off fresh mint and parsley while cooking!

Other Easy-to-grow Vegetables

- **Spring onions and radishes:** sow in pots or in the ground.
- **Potatoes:** plant February–March in potato bags part-filled with compost; when green shoots appear, cover with more compost.
- **Peas:** perfect for the UK, as they like cooler weather. Fresh-picked peas are sweet and tasty.
- **Tomatoes:** quick and super-simple to grow, they can be sown in hanging baskets, pots or window boxes – either from seeds or shoots.
- **Beetroot:** vividly colourful and unbelievably good for you! Boiled or steamed beetroot is versatile: ideal for chopping into salads, eating with other vegetables or in risotto.

> *I can think of no better form of personal involvement in the cure of the environment than that of gardening. A person who is growing a garden… is improving a piece of the world.*
> **Wendell Berry**
> *The Art of the Commonplace: The Agrarian Essays*

Guerrilla Gardening

A few years ago I lived in a part of London called Elephant and Castle, a true inner-city area. Although it isn't far from some beautiful parks and the River Thames, the neighbourhood itself has some of the highest-density social housing in Europe, a large and traffic-choked roundabout and a reputation for mean streets. Despite the less-than-leafy surroundings, a local man named Richard Reynolds was becoming known as the Guerrilla Gardener.

Guerrilla gardening is defined on Wikipedia as 'the act of gardening on land that the gardeners do not have the legal rights to utilize, such as an abandoned site, an area that is not being cared for, or private property'. In Elephant, Reynolds and his fellow guerrillas would plant up small patches of grass (often at night), transforming housing estates and shabby streets into a riot of wild flowers. Imagine the delight of seeing sprigs of daffodils sprouting beside the tube station, violets growing in the middle of the death-trap roundabout or herbs filling the previously derelict subway.

What started as 'illicit cultivation around London' has developed into a 'war against neglect and scarcity of public space as a place to grow things'.

Rewilding Britain

For decades conservationists have been working on rewilding projects across the world, from the reintroduction of wolf packs to Yellowstone Park to cheetahs in India – and now it's taking off in Britain too. A movement is underway to reintroduce long-gone species and to revert some of the UK's landscapes to a wilder state.

As well as reintroducing extinct species, rewilding schemes have been reclaiming and restoring river courses, forests, moorland and bogs, and planting thousands of native trees, flowers and rare grasses. Remote wetlands that once contained a wide variety of flora and fauna are being returned to nature.

In 2009, beavers were reintroduced to the Knapdale Forest in Scotland. A native species to the UK, they were hunted to extinction in the sixteenth century. By modifying their surroundings through coppicing and, in some cases, damming, beavers create ponds and wetlands which attract other species, provide a food source to others and can even help to improve water quality. For this reason, they are known as a 'keystone' species.

Like most environmental initiatives, rewilding is controversial. Should we be interfering in the ecosystem? Sceptics raise concerns over how the Eurasian lynx will fare in modern Britain and whether we really want wolves roaming the Scottish Highlands. From a primal perspective, it's wonderful to imagine indigenous species returning to their original habitat, but of course it's not that simple. This kind of ecological intervention has to be carefully considered, in order not to further disrupt nature's delicate balance.

Rewild Your Home

Every little helps, and we can all encourage biodiversity in and around our homes. You can start by planting wild flowers in your garden or window boxes to encourage birds and bees, or just leave water and seeds out for them. And, every day, open the windows to let the outside world – and fresh air – into your home.

Houses and offices may appear to be sealed off from obvious fumes and pollutants, but indoor air quality is still a major health concern. Stagnant indoor environments allow pollutants to build up and stick around; heating, insulation and air conditioning systems add to the foreign substances that we're breathing in. Furnishings, upholstery, synthetic building materials, and cleaning products in homes and offices can emit a variety of toxic compounds, like formaldehyde. Pollen, bacteria, moulds and external contaminants like car exhaust can find their way into buildings, and are worse in small or poorly ventilated spaces.

If you're not convinced, look at the harmful effects of asbestos. Although concerns had been raised about this widely used insulating material as early as the 1900s, it wasn't until the 1970s that the extent of the danger was publicly acknowledged. Exposure to asbestos in mines, factories, industry, transport, buildings, homes and schools has been linked to painful diseases including lung conditions, lung disease, pulmonary fibrosis and cancers such as mesothelioma.

Asbestos is an extreme example, but living and working in spaces full of air contaminants and lacking decent ventilation can cause 'sick building syndrome', leading to headaches, dizziness, nausea, and eye, ear and nose irritation.

Getting Primal Indoors

Adding potted plants to a room has been shown to reduce the amount of air particulates – and there's no doubt that greener, plant-filled air is cleaner. NASA scientists have found that plants actually make people feel better. Hospital patients with plants in their rooms are found to have lower blood pressure and stress levels, and feel more positive. Indoor plants also keep you alert and reduce mental fatigue.

Pot plants help to purify the atmosphere. The following are fast-growing, hardy and easily available:

- spider plants
- ficus/weeping fig
- peace lily
- bamboo palm
- aloe vera
- golden pothos.

There's something satisfyingly primal about growing things: however ambitious or simple your indoor horticulture, plants will raise your spirits and improve your atmosphere. They look great, smell great and give you a sense of achievement. Pruning, watering, even the odd spot of leaf-polishing – looking after plants is fun. After all, they're green, clean, *and* good for your mental and physical health.

> **❝** *I'm not running for sainthood. I just happen to think that in life we need to be like the farmer, who puts back into the soil what he takes out.* **❞**
> **Paul Newman**

Smarter Cars

We live in an age of gas-guzzling vehicles. Fuelling our transport, from planes to trains to lorries to individual cars, is one of the greatest energy demands of our time. While walking and cycling are good alternatives in and around towns and cities, for those travelling longer distances, or living in rural areas, driving can be unavoidable.

However, there are solutions. Low-emission vehicles cover a range of greener machines, including electric cars, cars that are part electric and part powered by petrol or diesel, range extenders and plug-ins and hybrids. The significant growth in sales of these vehicles is encouraging but, as with all green technology, it's a chicken-and-egg situation. Until cars have a longer battery life, and until there are more places to plug them in for recharging, take-up will be limited. It's still far easier to fill your tank with petrol than it is to recharge your smart car. Enlightened entrepreneurs, such as the founder of Tesla cars, Elon Musk, are leading the way, but we need much wider investment, and infrastructure in and around our towns and cities to encourage a wider take-up.

At an individual level, there are positive changes we can all make. Limiting individual car usage is the priority, using public transport where possible, and cutting down on flying. We also have to be prepared to make compromises in how and where we travel: perhaps making fewer journeys, and maybe sharing cars. The concept of carpooling has never quite taken off – it's a shame to still see so many individually occupied vehicles making the same trips, which could easily be shared, day-in day-out.

Of course, we need to move from place to place, but there are more primal ways of getting around. The less we pollute the air, the pleasanter it is to be outside. One of the most primal of all pleasures is eating outdoors: try it if you can! I often have a morning espresso on my balcony to gather my thoughts for the day ahead. You can always throw on a fleece and/or shelter under an umbrella, or construct a small gazebo. You could take your morning toast into the garden, or pack a picnic for a nearby meadow, forest or beach. As long as you have a really good coat (a ski jacket is ideal) and it's not raining, you can grab the occasional meal outdoors pretty much year-round. Fresh air stimulates the appetite and, especially in winter, fish and chips taste great by the British seaside. If you're stuck in an office, take your sandwiches to the local park: notice the flowers, feed the birds, and boost your vitamin D intake. When eating at work, try al fresco rather than al desko.

If it's really too wet or cold to get outside, try to arrange your desk or your kitchen table so it has a view of the outdoors. Letting a little daylight into your home will enliven those dreary household chores and lift your primal spirits.

Go Eco

When rewilding your inside and outside spaces, and purifying your air, it's worth thinking about what else goes on in your home: specifically washing and cleaning.

You don't need a lecture about all the ecologically friendly detergents out there – but consider using them. They cost a little more, but it really is a 'little': my monthly outlay on eco-friendly products (washing-up liquid, non-bio laundry liquid and household cleaner) is probably the equivalent extra cost of a couple of take-away coffees.

It *is* worth it. The products are made from plant-based and mineral ingredients, they're non-toxic to your skin and completely bio-degradable, which means that they absorb back into nature. They smell good and clean properly, and the 'plantplastic' bottles are 100 per cent recyclable. In the same way, use recycled kitchen roll and lavatory paper wherever you can. Synthetic air fresheners are full of unnecessary, potentially toxic, ingredients. The best way to air your home is to open windows and keep plenty of plants.

Most mainstream household products contain bleach, sodium hypochlorite, hypochlorite and chlorine. However, chlorine is toxic, and it can affect the immune system, thyroid and respiratory system. Instead of relying on harsh commercial cleaning products, get into the habit of using natural alternatives. There are many safe, cheap options, including vinegar, lemon, borax and tea tree oil. These will do everything from scouring pots and pans to removing limescale and giving you sparkling streak-free windows. Bicarbonate of soda is an excellent all-purpose cleaner. Dilute it in warm water for cleaning or put a small dish in the fridge overnight to banish smells (check www. ewg.org for more suggestions).

Clear white vinegar is a versatile cleaner. It gives great results and cheap supermarket versions are fine. Use it:

- to clean lime deposits from hard water on sinks – wrap a few paper towels tightly around taps and fixtures, pour vinegar onto the towels and leave for ten to 30 minutes

- to remove hard water build-up in the kettle – fill it with vinegar and leave for 30 minutes; rinse well

- to clean drains by pouring half a cup of baking soda down first, followed by half a cup of vinegar, and then cover the drain for ten minutes; turn the tap on and rinse through thoroughly

- to clean a coffee maker – pour half a pot of vinegar and run it through the cycle; then run one or two cycles of plain water

- for windows and mirrors – combine two parts water, one part vinegar and a drop of washing-up liquid

- to clean and freshen up your dishwasher – add a cup of vinegar to a dishwashing cycle

- to remove stains and oxidation from stainless steel and copper cookware – use a solution of two tablespoons of vinegar mixed with two teaspoons of table salt

- for cleaning up pet accidents on the carpet and also to get rid of fleas – make a spray of one part vinegar to six parts water, and spray on rugs, floors and carpets.

Dry-cleaning

The chemicals used in dry-cleaning tend to be very harsh: try to limit your exposure. 'Dry clean-only' labels are often used as a cover-all by manufacturers, but in fact most items of clothing can be safely washed by hand or even in a washing machine. Use cool water, or a gentle 30-degree cycle, and they should be fine. If something is precious, or highly decorated or embellished – say a wedding dress or evening dress with sequins – it probably will need professional cleaning. Always remove the plastic covering and hang up clothes after dry-cleaning, to air out the chemicals.

Primal Working

As you become more primal and green at home, you'll probably notice ways to be more primal at work too. Pot plants are ideal in office environments. Not only does the greenery enliven drab spaces, they also refresh stale atmospheres. Some offices these days are sealed, air-conditioned spaces, especially the glass tower blocks: you may not be allowed to open the windows, but no one can object to a few pot plants! Watering and tending also help to break up the working day, and give colleagues a shared interest.

Remember those office reminders about wasting less paper: 'Do you really need to print this email?' It took us a while to realise that printing out everything *isn't* necessary and it wastes precious natural resources. The digital revolution has made paperless offices a reality, with the majority of work being done on-screen, and emailed back and forth without the need for endless, wasteful reams of paper.

It's concerning, therefore, to see the development of 3-D printers. If they become as ubiquitous as predicted – in every home so we can print anything from toothbrushes to kitchen gadgets and children's toys – we must be careful not to become as thoughtless and casual about plastic wastage as we have been, for decades, about paper.

Pause For Thought

In Bristol city centre, some of the public bins have two sections, one for recyclables and one for non-recyclables. The non-recyclable bin is labelled 'LANDFILL' instead of general waste. It's a subtle shift of emphasis, but clever: it makes you think about where the majority of our refuse actually ends up. Do we really want all that trash being tipped into our green and pleasant lands?

Do No Harm

Ahimsa is the Buddhist principle of doing no harm. The literal meaning of the Sanskrit term is 'non-injury' and 'non-killing'. It implies the total avoidance of any kind of harming of living creatures not only by deeds, but also by words and in thoughts. This core principle of non-violence is found at the heart of Jainism and Hinduism, as well as Buddhism.

The Indian independence leader and lawyer Mahatma Gandhi promoted the principle of Ahimsa in all areas of life, especially politics. His non-violent resistance movement known as *satyagraha* had an immense impact in the 1930s and 1940s, and influenced other civil rights leaders such as Martin Luther King.

Some Jain followers take Ahimsa to an extreme degree. Their vow to do no harm extends to every living thing, no matter how tiny. Strict Jains do not go out at night, for example, when they are more likely to step upon small insects or worms. Eating honey is strictly outlawed, as it would amount to violence against the bees. Some even consider words to be a form of harm, and keep a cloth to ritually cover their mouth, as a reminder not to allow violence in their speech.

Following the Ahimsa belief system to these extremes is clearly not feasible for most of us. For example, as a vegetarian I dislike the idea of harming other animals, but I accept that I cannot avoid treading on insects. However, the principle of Ahimsa raises some interesting ideas for our primal journey; specifically, how we co-exist with others and how we might walk more lightly on this Earth.

If you find the concept of Ahimsa interesting, I highly recommend Philip Roth's 1997 novel, *American Pastoral*.

> **Alex, 52:** We recently moved to a very 'alternative' area of Bristol called Stokes Croft, and all our neighbours are militant recyclers. When we first arrived, I felt anxious every time Friday came around: was it the week for food waste or green waste, mixed recyclables or non-recyclables? After a few months I've got used to the complicated bin collection calendars, and I no longer have to smuggle the bins out under cover of darkness. Yes, it takes a bit more thought – but so what? The amount of packaging and plastic we generate is a scandal, and most of it is entirely unnecessary. I'm loving the new green lifestyle, and finally feel like I'm part of a community.

To me, there is no downside to this way of living. There's a reason why renewables are referred to as 'clean' energy: it's self-evidently cleaner not to pollute the planet which sustains us. In the past few centuries of industrialisation we've already done untold damage: there are rainforests we'll never replant, coral reefs we'll never regrow and carbon dioxide we can never take back. But our world is surprisingly resilient: according to a 2010 UN report, even the infamous 'hole in the ozone' is regenerating itself and the ozone could be back to full strength by the middle of the century.

If it was possible to take action on aerosols and CFCs, why not other pollutants? If we can buy, consume and waste less, with little hardship to ourselves – and manifold benefits – why wouldn't we? Why *not* pledge to treat this Earth with a little more respect?

Our Primal Planet

Adopting a primal attitude to the environment, to some extent, requires you to put your fingers in your ears and ignore the nihilistic view that nothing we do has any impact. It calls upon you to believe in the power of the individual and the community to make a difference. Even if you can't save the planet, isn't it worth making your local neighbourhood a more pleasant place to live?

Look at it another way: what happens if we don't bother to change anything? If we keep on pumping CO_2 into the atmosphere, filling the oceans with plastic and the earth with our trash, drilling and fracking, emitting and warming. How many more species will become extinct? How many more rainforests will we lose? How much more erosion of coastlines, melting of glaciers and rising of sea levels will we experience? How many more of our fellow citizens will be driven from their homes by extreme weather and natural disasters?

Primal living isn't only about limiting the damage we do; it's also about conserving, preserving a way of life, a natural landscape, and a cultural and linguistic heritage. When we lose wildlife, we lose language and poetry too. Over the past decade the following words have disappeared from the *Junior Oxford English Dictionary*: *acorn*, *buttercup* and *conker*. They have made way for words such as *broadband*, *blog* and *download*. The word *Blackberry* is listed, but it is defined as a phone rather than a fruit. What a shame that the language of new technology cannot exist alongside the more primal pleasures of life.

If we can conserve our wetlands, if we can nurture our endangered species, why wouldn't we? Why not plant wild flowers on our motorway verges? If work and effort are worth anything, aren't they worth devoting to such fragile life forms? Humans may be thoughtless, too often, but we are not stupid. It's not beyond us to find a way to link our desire for constant economic growth and consumption with a greener world: to make the ever-increasing demands for energy a force for good.

The good news is that creating a more primal world around you can be incredibly fun. Starting a compost heap is ace (anyone for a wormery?), taking a cloth bag with you to the supermarket is easy, and mending, swapping and up-cycling offer hours of harmless amusement. When is the last time you darned a hole in your socks? Everyone has to start somewhere…

Can we leave a world for future generations in which both *buttercup* and *broadband* have a place in our dictionary? If not, in the words of the great US conservationist Aldo Leopold, 'I am glad I will not be young in a future without wilderness.'

Chapter 14

Primal Spirituality

Would you describe yourself as 'religious'? If not, what about 'spiritual'? Do you ever feel *there must be more to life than this* – even if you're not sure what that *more* might be?

Spirituality in the twenty-first century is a thorny issue. An alien landing on Earth might be forgiven for thinking that those shiny rectangular devices we carry around contain some vital life force, without which we would wither and die. They might assume that those screens we're glued to are relaying instructions to us from some mysterious higher power. The ubiquity of our smartphones, laptops and tablets might indicate membership of some kind of cult: as quickly as we've cast off organised religion in the twentieth century, we have embraced media, capitalism and digital technology.

There's no doubt we're attached, if not addicted, to that virtual reality. Yet we're not entirely shallow: whether we class ourselves as believers or non-believers, most of us still want to believe that our existence has meaning. We naturally look for significance in our lives: we want to understand what we're doing here and what happens to us when we die. We seek reassurance from our existential anxiety in the thought that there may be something beyond...

This search for meaning is when we're at our most primal, our most human. We're surrounded by miracles and tragedies: in every newborn baby or bereavement we face profound, unanswerable questions about life and death, love and loss. Unlike animals, it's not enough for us just to sleep, eat, repeat. At a more primal level, we want to understand why we live and why we die. Even if we're not religious, we still have questions about *what it all means.*

Religious or Spiritual?

Are these terms interchangeable or are they diametrically opposed? Many people who consider themselves spiritual feel quite hostile to organised religion, and many formal churchgoers dismiss those who follow alternative belief systems and call themselves spiritual. It's a shame there isn't more tolerance and respect between believers, no matter where they find their inner peace, what they believe or how they practise. After all, both ideologies share a sense that there is something beyond this physical world, whatever that *something* might be.

Church attendance in the UK declined sharply throughout the twentieth century and continues to fall. The 2014 British Social Attitudes survey found that 58.4 per cent of the population never attend religious services and only 13.1 per cent of people report going to a service once a week or more. Other surveys have put the UK attendance rate as low as six per cent. Global statistics also vary: a Gallup Poll in 2004 put regular church attendance at around 39 per cent in the United States, 12 per cent in France and 7.5 per cent in Australia.

Those steadily decreasing rates suggest that many of us find organised religion off-putting or simply irrelevant to our lives. This decline is at its fastest among young people: in the 2011 UK census, nearly 32 per cent of under-25s said that they had no religious belief.

Spiritual But Not Religious

Perhaps rather than actively rejecting the notion of God, the reality is that we've been brought up without it. We don't go with friends or family to church on a Sunday morning simply because it was never part of our upbringing. Sure, churches are picturesque – they give a sense of history and heritage to our towns – but we don't *use* them. We pop into foreign cathedrals, mosques or temples when we're on holiday or travelling abroad. But in our busy daily lives the majority of us have no use for these holy spaces and no time for quiet reflection.

We may not have time to reflect, but that doesn't mean that we don't need to. The search for meaning never goes away. In the gap left by organised religion, increasingly people are self-identifying as 'spiritual'. It's an imprecise term, with a wide range of meanings and experiences: from the sense that there's something beyond the humdrum, a yearning for a deeper connection to the world around us, or intense moments of awe and wonder, even transcendence. Perhaps the term 'spiritual' stands for those things which we can't put into words. Often characterised as a pick-and-mix approach to contemporary culture, spiritualism encompasses alternative therapies, meditation, yoga, reflexology and homeopathy, and belief systems such as humanism, paganism and even fortune-telling.

I'm not formally religious. Like many, however, I find that the liturgy and the ritual speak to something within me, at an emotional, even spiritual, level. When I make time to attend church, once or twice a month, I feel peaceful for the rest of the day, less frazzled and frantic. The very act of communion with others – shaking hands with strangers and wishing them peace, partaking in the mystery of bread and wine – transforms a normal Sunday into something rather special. There aren't many places these days where you can walk into someone else's close-knit group and be welcomed, without any questions asked. It feels elemental and primal, sitting peacefully in contemplation with others.

But how much longer will churches exist? Philip Larkin's poem 'Church Going' predicts a time when these houses of God will be obsolete. The narrator is passing through an unfamiliar part of England and stops to visit a deserted church. As he stands there, he wonders:

> 66 *When churches fall completely out of use*
> *What we shall turn them into...* 99

Going to church these days, one can't help but feel this time has come. Most churchgoers now are elderly: when they die, who will fill our places of worship?

It's well known that people who have strong social networks live longer, healthier lives. Research shows that those who attend church also rate their levels of happiness more highly. Being part of a community helps to prevent isolation and loneliness, which make us mentally and physically unwell. Religious attendance bolsters people's sense of belonging, and has a beneficial effect on their physical and psychological well-being.

At the end of every service, the vicar at my local church reminds his flock to 'give thanks for the abundance which surrounds us, and pray for all those who live in poverty or hunger'. But why does this need to be called 'prayer'? Would it be possible to live like this anyway, with or without religious belief? Primal spirituality is about taking these traditional values of generosity, charity and kindness, and embedding them into your everyday life.

Everyday Goodness

I recently heard a story about a food bank which had been set up at the exit of a large supermarket. A middle-aged man, well-dressed and holding the keys to an expensive Audi, was leaving the store, pushing a trolley filled with six shopping bags. He stopped at the food bank collection point and unloaded five bags, keeping one for himself. He'd been through rough times himself, he explained to the volunteer.

Everything about this man's outward appearance suggested a wealthy city slicker, probably in banking or public relations, but his behaviour told a different story. His actions weren't about ostentatious do-gooding or charitable work, nor was he seeking public recognition. He was just being a compassionate human being, choosing to care about others. You don't have to be religious to have good, human values.

A Force for Good or Evil?

Religious extremism is a sad and horrifying fact of our times. We are witnessing the rise of groups such as the so-called 'Islamic State' in Syria and Iraq, recruiting foreign fighters for global jihad and war on the West, and Boko Haram in Nigeria, kidnapping children and young women to use as killers and sex slaves. According to the Global Terrorism Index, terrorism increased 80 per cent from 2013 to 2014, with an estimated 32,658 people killed in attacks around the world.

With the 24–7 news cycle, social media propaganda, podcasts in multiple languages and every terrible beheading going viral, some consider religion itself to be the root of all this evil. But it's nothing new: atrocities have been committed in the name of God since the time of the Crusades and well before. I would even hesitate to use the term 'religion' in the context of such inhumanity: it seems an insult to all decent Muslims, Christians and other believers.

Such evil – committed in the name of God or Allah – must be weighed against the good that ordinary people, devout, agnostic or atheist, do every day. There is a handwritten sign on the door of an old church in my neighbourhood: 'We aspire to cherish all, regardless of marital, social or economic status, sexual orientation, race or gender.' That's a doctrine we can all sign up to, surely – believers or not. Staying primal means believing in mankind and never giving up on human beings as a force for good.

Modern Faith

The Buddha declared 2,500 years ago: 'I teach suffering, its origin, cessation and path. That's all I teach.' Buddhism has ancient roots but enduring modern relevance. The philosophy has spread from a solitary order in a remote area of India in the fifth century BC, via 1950s America where Zen was all the rage with the Beat Generation, to the global mindfulness movement of today. The Buddha's teachings are based around Four Noble Truths.

- The truth of suffering (Dukkha): suffering is an inescapable part of life. Human life includes struggle, anguish and pain.

- The truth of the cause of suffering (Samudaya): all suffering stems from desire, *tanhā*. The three roots of evil are greed, ignorance and hatred that arise in our minds – our own desires to avoid the difficulties that we encounter. Attachment to positive, negative and neutral sensations and thoughts is the cause of suffering.

- The truth of freedom from suffering (Nirodha): all attachments, sensation and thoughts – whether pleasurable, unpleasant or neutral – cause suffering. In order to end this cycle of suffering, we must respond differently and free ourselves from attachment. We must end the anger, greed and delusion that prevent us from knowing and understanding the truth.

The truth of the path that leads to the end of suffering (Magga): we can achieve happiness, virtue and nirvana through positive action, and by following the Noble Eightfold Path, including living ethically, and avoiding killing, stealing, lying, drinking or sexual misconduct. We must cultivate discipline, act decently, and practise mindfulness and meditation. Only then are we liberated from the cycle of death and rebirth, dissatisfaction, clinging, and craving.

Mastering mindfulness and meditation is a vital part of the Buddhist journey towards nirvana.

Meditation and Mindfulness

The Buddha taught that meditation and mindfulness provided space in people's busy lives to develop understanding and help them to live well. Meditation calms the mind. Sitting quietly provides the opportunity to think deeply, and to see why it is better to live ethically and why attachment to things, people and ideas leads to pain. Buddhist meditation practices are wide-ranging, from silence to chanting.

In modern humanism, and in the increasing popularity of yoga, meditation and mindfulness – even in the environmental movement – we can see the resurgence of a new kind of spirituality or faith. Whatever we call it, and wherever we find it, these practices are forms of communion with ourselves and the world around us.

Meditation is a valuable skill for life. Just sitting quietly, breathing in and out, you begin to create a cycle of relaxation: inhaling oxygen and exhaling tension.

Try this practical breathing exercise.

- Make sure you're comfortable: loosen any belts or tight zips, and sit in a chair that supports your neck and head, or lie down flat.

- Place your arms along the chair arms, or flat on the floor or bed, slightly apart from your body, with palms facing upwards.

- If you're sitting down, keep your legs uncrossed. If you're lying down, stretch out your legs, keeping them hip-width apart.

⬧ Begin to inhale and exhale slowly, filling your lungs with air and maintaining a regular rhythm.

⬧ Breathe in through your nose and out through your mouth, counting 1-2-3 on the inhale and 1-2-3 on the exhale. Keep going for five minutes, or until you start to feel calm.

This simple exercise can be repeated anytime, anywhere. It's effective for reducing stress or tension, and will help you to stay calm during periods of anxiety, for example before giving a speech. It's also the ideal way to prepare for some primal, positive meditation.

Now you've mastered deep breathing, but the mental aspect of meditation can be much harder. You know the struggle: *how do I empty my mind? How do I stop myself from worrying, obsessing and stressing? How do I get rid of these repetitive thoughts? Why am I thinking about dinner when I should be meditating? Am I doing this right – when do I start to feel spiritual?*

The answer to the last question, of course, is that you don't. Or at least you don't by consciously trying. Meditation is a way of learning to rise above the anxieties and irritations of everyday life. It doesn't prevent them from occurring, but it gives your overactive mind a place to go when they do. Meditation, practised regularly, allows you to find that distance between what you're thinking and who you are.

This is where mindfulness comes in: learning to observe the thoughts as they arise without hanging on to them, and to let them pass through your mind, almost like clouds. My yoga teacher likens those repetitive, obtrusive thoughts we all have to an eager, overexcited puppy who keeps jumping up: 'You acknowledge it, and gently push it away.' So you allow those thoughts to come and go.

Mindfulness training has seen a huge surge in popularity in the twenty-first century. With roots in Buddhism and ancient Eastern traditions, it also incorporates very modern cultural beliefs and advances in neuroscience, and physiological, cognitive and social developments. The benefits of meditation have been known for thousands of years; mindfulness is a combination of the spiritual, the physical and the scientific.

According to a study in *The Lancet* (April 2015), meditation and mindfulness help to prevent the recurrence of depression. They can also reduce the risk of heart attack by 11 per cent and stroke by up to 15 per cent (American Heart Association). Meditation could also be good for your skin: a study from Harvard University found that meditation results in 'cortical thickness' in the parts of the brain that reduce stress and anxiety. This in turn reduces inflammation of the skin that causes ageing. If you're new to meditation, why not start by following a guided meditation on YouTube or downloading an app? Headspace and Buddhify are among the most popular apps and are ideal for beginners.

Ten minutes every morning is manageable for most of us, and a deeply primal, grounding way to start the day. Sit in silence and breathe rhythmically, inhaling through your nose on a count of three, and then exhaling on a count of three. This will calm your nervous system and heart rate, which in turn will bring your thoughts under control.

Everyday Mindfulness

Mindfulness is exactly what it sounds like: a way of being more aware, or 'mindful', of the world around you. The opposite, being mindless, is like living on automatic pilot: you eat an entire pack of biscuits, or drive a familiar journey, without even registering what you've done.

It's easy to incorporate mindfulness into your daily life: by slowing down, focusing and taking time over the task in hand. It doesn't need to be profound or complicated – in fact, the simpler the better. You can practise mindfulness when walking to the shops, loading the laundry or chopping vegetables, simply by doing them with attention. When walking, look around you, feel the air on your face, focus on the pavement or the grass you're walking on, slow down and then quicken your pace, swing your arms. You can apply the same principle in the kitchen: just focus on the vegetables you're chopping: the deep colour of beetroot, the tiny trees on each stem of broccoli, and the bumps and creases of every carrot.

I think of these as little moments of 'noticing' in the everyday, moments when we zone out of the mental chatter in our brains and zoom in on the physical world which surrounds us. It's a way of pressing pause, of paying attention to the quirks, colours, sounds and scents of our environment. Focusing fully on anything from knobbly vegetables to uneven paving stones to damp grass can be a deeply spiritual experience: it is tuning into the primal sensation of what it means to be alive.

Primal, Mindful Eating

Mindful eating is powerful because it helps you to slow down and notice what you're actually putting in your mouth. How does it taste? How does it make you feel? Overeating (and other forms of disordered eating) often comes from mixing up emotions with hunger or cravings, burying difficult feelings in food or simply not registering what we're putting in our mouths. Mealtimes are an excellent opportunity for practising mindfulness. Eating with attention and care, as opposed to shovelling down the same old sandwich while fiddling online, is rewarding. Here are a few primal pointers for mindful eating.

- **Avoid eating in front of your computer screen, or while making a phone call or walking down the street.** At home, turn off the TV and lay the table. Make meals a pleasurable occasion: use a plate, knife and fork.

- **Slow down:** take time to stop and taste the food. Put your cutlery down between bites and chew each mouthful properly.

- **Keep sipping:** sip water between mouthfuls to aid digestion and keep you hydrated. Drink water throughout the day, so as not to confuse thirst with hunger.

- **Cook mindfully:** enjoy the process of preparing meals, even if you live alone. Be mentally present and savour the aromas. Chopping, stirring and seasoning are very meditative.

- **Pole position:** place healthy food where you can see it and be easily tempted. Keep fresh fruit on your desk and fresh vegetables at the front of the fridge.

🍃 **Experiment:** taste new foods, buy cookery books, shop at markets and try new recipes. Doing these things keeps your diet varied and avoids mindless eating ruts.

🍃 **Check your dining companions:** we tend to unconsciously eat in tandem, so be mindful of how others influence your habits. Focus on what *your* body needs, rather than what others are eating.

🍃 **Eat more fibre:** this helps to regulate your blood sugar levels, avoiding cravings and crashes.

🍃 **Eat the colours of the rainbow:** fresh, healthy food – think carrots, tomatoes, beetroot and broccoli – is bursting with essential nutrients. A colourful diet tends to be more balanced.

🍃 **Don't eat when you're in an emotional state.** Sit with your feelings rather than fleeing them. Determine whether you are hungry or bored, angry or upset. Developing self-awareness helps to prevent mindless eating.

Exercise Your Spirituality

For many nowadays spirituality comes in a physical form – yoga or meditation, for example – and with good reason. There is an overwhelming consensus that physical activity is beneficial for our emotional and cognitive well-being. The Royal College of Psychiatrists report that 'for mild depression, physical activity can be as good as antidepressants or psychological treatments like cognitive behavioural therapy'. There are many reasons why exercise is so brilliant for our heads.

🍃 Activity affects certain brain chemicals associated with mood, particularly dopamine and serotonin. Brain cells use these chemicals to communicate with each other, so they affect your thinking and behaviour.

🍃 Exercise seems to reduce harmful changes in the brain caused by stress.

▸ Exercise helps you to escape from stressors at work/home – it literally gives you headspace.

▸ Exercise helps you to sleep, gives you energy, and boosts your confidence and self-esteem.

▸ Exercise gives you a sense of control over your life. It helps you to feel capable, healthy and strong. It's also very uplifting.

▸ Finally – if you can get outdoors, do! Exercising in nature has profound soothing and restorative qualities.

We're hard-wired for activity and movement, and this is why exercise makes us feel good. Our primal predecessors had to move to get food, water and shelter – and many people in the world still do. Activity reminds us that we're human and takes us back to our primal roots.

The Yoga Explosion

It's easy to scoff at superficial happy-clappy spirituality. There is plenty of fashionable faith floating around these days, from the wearing of bindis as a style statement to the immaculately clad yoga fashionistas to the profound Sanskrit tattoos which routinely adorn many wrists and ankles. However, when practised authentically – not expertly, but simply with humility and awareness – yoga can be transformative.

It's this challenging, authentic element of yoga which has touched practitioners in every corner of the Earth. In June 2015 the United Nations marked the first ever International Yoga Day. The roots of yoga and meditation go back thousands of years, and millions of humans through many centuries have found it helpful in their lives. Whether you practise yoga for physical fitness, to help with aches and pains, to stay supple, to counteract stress and anxiety, to cope with tough times or sadness, to get headspace in a busy schedule, to challenge yourself or simply for the pure enjoyment, it can be a powerful tool for getting in touch with your primal self.

Staying in a Difficult Place

Although social media is awash with pictures of lithe yoginis executing complicated poses in stunning settings, there's far more to yoga than that. The benefits for body and soul are genuine. Yoga develops mental and emotional strength, as well as physical flexibility. It isn't just about bending and stretching and holding a pose; it's about staying in an unaccustomed position. Literally: learning to be in a difficult place.

Many asanas are uncomfortable, especially at first. Apply this to your life – to relationships or work, say – and it becomes a profound learning process. In yoga, you learn how to breathe through discomfort, how to be patient and hold on, how to shift your weight to make things work. Sitting and meditating, noticing itches or twinges: can you live with it? And if not, what can you do to overcome it? Most of all, you're practising how to find balance.

This process takes place every time you return to the yoga mat. How does your mind react when your body is trying to do something difficult? And when you fail or fall, how do you react? Can you rediscover that outer equilibrium, and restore your inner calm? Just as in life, in yoga you find your balance and lose it, and have to find it again. Yoga is a process of trusting and adjusting, breathing and balance.

There are thousands of great yoga apps out there, tailored to every level of ability and fitness. You can do as much or as little as you want: a full workout or simply a few relaxing asanas at the end of a long day. They're ideal for when you're travelling: you can fit in a few bends and stretches in your hotel room, at the back of the plane, wherever you might be...

Stella Ralfini, a yoga teacher, reiki healer and author of *Chakra Psychology*, who lives near me in London, captures the essence of yoga:

❝ Many imagine yoga is mainly for the spiritually inclined, so let's put an end to that myth. Yoga doesn't care what you are, whether you eat meat, smoke cigarettes or enjoy vodka on the rocks – although most people who embrace yoga find they start dropping things they do to excess without realizing it. When taught correctly, yoga has the power to get into your mind. This is achieved by opening the chakras through certain body postures and breathing techniques. Yoga is more than an exercise form. Yoga fuses the body with the mind and soul so that you are able to stretch the body. ❞

Yoga is also ageless. Most sports are age-sensitive: few top flight tennis players or footballers are still playing beyond 35, and ballerinas face a similarly short shelf life. For me, one of the most beautiful aspects of yoga is the people who practise it, of all ages. I take classes with the most agile and serene women in their 50s, 70s and even 90s. Because guess what? Flexibility and grace don't disappear, not if you're practising regularly. Quite the opposite: a well-trained yoga body retains its inner firmness and agility, no matter how old or wrinkled the skin may become.

Yoga is not individually competitive like other sports. It's about 'you' working with 'you' to improve your own practice. Yoga is introspective in a positive sense: it's about finding peace within, rather than comparing yourself with the world outside.

American and Dutch scientists have found that yoga can be as effective at combating heart disease as traditional aerobic exercise. It helps with high blood pressure, depression, stress, lower back pain and osteoarthritis. It develops strength and balance, eases tension, and keeps you flexible, so it's ideal for people of all shapes, sizes, ages and fitness levels.

Which Kind?

There are many different types of yoga: some dynamic and physically challenging and others more focused on spirituality, relaxation or breath work. If you're a beginner, you should try out a few different classes to see which suits your temperament. Also, find a yoga instructor you enjoy working with, explain what you're looking for and ask their advice.

Hatha yoga: focuses on slow and gentle movements. Hatha refers to the physical aspects of yoga, the asanas; hatha yoga is good for beginners, as it covers the basic asanas. It's also ideal to wind down at the end of a long day if you have an active, stressful job.

Vinyasa yoga: also known as dynamic flow, or just flow, this is the most popular form of yoga in America. Poses flow from one to the next, so it's an excellent physical workout. It's more suitable for intermediate to advanced level, rather than beginners.

Kundalini yoga: this is all about awakening the energy in your spine (kundalini refers to the root chakra), with many poses focusing on the lower spine and 'core' area. It also incorporates meditation, chanting and breath work.

Ashtanga yoga: also known as power yoga, Ashtanga is physically demanding – best suited for more advanced yoga practitioners or those looking to push their body.

Iyengar yoga: focuses on correct alignment, using props such as blocks, harnesses, straps and cushions. This makes Iyengar good for beginners, or for those doing yoga for physical therapy or in rehabilitation from injury.

Anusara yoga: derived from Iyengar, within the Hatha school of yoga. Founded in 1997 by John Friend, Anusara incorporates many 'heart-opening' poses like backbends. Anusara is based around three core principles (attitude, alignment and action), focal points and energy loops.

Jivamukti yoga: the celebrity one! Jivamukti means 'liberation while living'. It was founded in New York City in 1984, and is a philosophy and a lifestyle as much as a form of yoga. It combines vigorous Hatha and Vinyasa flow with chanting, music and scripture readings. Jivamukti incorporates physical, ethical and spiritual elements, as well as veganism, environmentalism and social activism.

Restorative yoga: simple poses, supported by pillows and bolsters. It focuses on relaxation, so it's ideal for unwinding at the end of a long day; also good for mental relaxation and learning how to quieten your mind.

Bikram yoga: the hot one! Created by Indian yogi Bikram Choudhury in the 1970s, Bikram is designed around a sequence of 26 yoga poses to stretch and strengthen the muscles, as well as compress and 'rinse' the organs of the body. The poses are done in a heated room – sometimes up to 40°C and 40 per cent humidity – to facilitate the release of toxins. Every Bikram class you go to, anywhere in the world, follows the same sequence of 26 poses.

Pranayama

In yogic science, breath is the thread which binds us to the body, *prana* meaning breath or life force. Breathing is a bridge between the conscious and the subconscious, an intangible link between the body, mind and spirit. The diaphragm is both a voluntary and an involuntary muscle: it keeps you breathing and alive when you're asleep, but you can control it when you're awake. Understanding the importance of breathing – or pranayama, the control or extension of this life force – is vital to meditation.

When your mind is clear and balanced, your breath is even and rhythmic. On the other hand, when your mind is nervous and tense, your breath is fast or irregular. The stronger your lungs and the steadier your breathing, the greater your energy and mental clarity.

Breathing is both a reminder of the fragility of being alive and a powerful way into meditation. A central focus of yoga and meditation is to make the unconscious conscious. Pranayama brings the breath and *prana* into consciousness.

Here's a simple breathing meditation to get you started.

- Sit cross-legged – somewhere warm, wearing loose comfortable clothing – with your spine comfortably erect.

- Rest your hands loosely on your thighs.

- With your face upturned, allow your focus to settle naturally between your eyes.

- Repeat this simple statement, either in your head or out loud: 'I'm not the body' on the inhale and 'I'm not even the mind' on the exhale.

- Repeat this 50 times, each time inhaling: 'I'm not the body' and exhaling 'I'm not even the mind'.

- Don't worry if your mind wanders or if you find it hard to keep control of your thoughts. Just keep bringing the focus back to your breath: inhaling and exhaling, repeating the mantra.

- Try this for a few minutes, gradually increasing to ten or 15 minutes. It takes practice, but you should find yourself getting lulled into a meditative state.

- Remember, this isn't about right or wrong. There is no such thing as a 'perfect' meditation: that's why it's called a practice!

Meditate for Happiness

Meditation isn't just about getting headspace in a busy schedule; research shows it can actually make you happier. The French-born Buddhist monk Matthieu Ricard has been called 'the happiest man in the world'. He lives in a Nepalese monastery with no heating, and has no property or income of his own. (He is a public speaker and author, but all profits from his work go to running a humanitarian NGO.)

Neuroscientists at the University of Wisconsin studied Ricard's brain while he was meditating and discovered more heightened activity in the regions associated with positive emotions than had ever been recorded in any scientific literature. The research suggested that meditating for a long period of time might have the potential capacity to alter the brain, or even train oneself in happiness.

According to Ricard, the secret is to meditate for 20 minutes a day, and to make a conscious decision to look on the bright side. He believes that just four weeks of 'caring mindfulness' meditation can have a powerful effect on our brains, and enhance our immune systems. 'Anyone can be the happiest man or woman in the world if you look for happiness in the right place.' Rather than despairing of the world – with its inequality, civil wars and refugee crises – Ricard focuses on the perfectibility of humanity. He claims that globally violence rates are falling and he sees signs of grass-roots solidarity everywhere. There is, he says, 'something in the air'.

We use the term 'happy' all the time, but what do we really mean by it? Happiness is rare and somehow intangible. It means something different to each person, and cannot be bought, earned or sold. It comes and goes, fleeting and precious.

Happiness may be a mystery, but there are steps you can take to make yourself more open to it. Positive thinking, awareness of others and mindful gratitude all contribute to a more receptive outlook. When you focus on your surroundings, the beauty of the natural world, the love and kindness of the people around you... Well, every day has the potential to be something special.

You can educate yourself about happiness, too. I recommend Hermann Hesse's short book *Siddhartha*. It takes only a few hours to read, and is very thought-provoking. Siddhartha is the privileged son of a Brahmin. He sets out on a spiritual journey in search of enlightenment. At the start of the book his goal is 'to become empty, to become empty of thirst, desire, dreams, pleasure and sorrow – to let the Self die. No longer to be Self, to experience the peace of an emptied heart, to experience pure thought.'

Siddhartha's journey leads him to reject all worldly goods, living in hunger, patience and deep meditation with other spiritual seekers, and then into the temptations of luxury, wealth and sexual pleasure. It's only after experiencing both extreme poverty and sensual riches that he's able to find what he is looking for. After many years of pain and searching, he finds peace and fulfilment.

If you're interested in Buddhism, this is a great place to start. Siddhartha eventually learns to love the world, despite all its sins and virtue, ugliness and beauty: 'to leave it as it is, to love it and be glad to belong to it'. Just as the Buddhist monk Ricard has inspired people around the world as a living embodiment of positivity and peace, Siddhartha has given many readers hope.

Primal Spirituality

Another example of positive spirituality is the Indian mystic, humanitarian and yogi Sadhguru Jaggi Vasudev, known to his thousands of followers simply as Sadhguru. With his white beard and flowing robes, Sadhguru radiates calm. His skill is making those ancient Eastern traditions accessible to everyone, whatever their background or spiritual beliefs.

He speaks powerfully about the nature of pain, for example: how and why do we, as individuals, experience pain? Given that war and famine are almost non-existent in the West, most of our suffering is mental – in effect, it's pain we inflict upon ourselves. Whatever our life circumstances – married or not married, having children or being childless, being too busy or being unemployed, excessive wealth or poverty – it all seems to make us miserable. He asked: why is this? Why does every human state have the capacity to cause us pain?

And why, when this unhappiness is happening to us, do we look outside ourselves for the solution? Why do we invariably try to change other people and external factors, when really we need to look inside and fix ourselves? Compare the moments of joy you had as child with the moments of joy you have now. As children, we weren't hung up on finding happiness or inner peace – we just had it. As adults, it's rare to have a single day completely free of stress, fear or anxiety.

All the progress of the past century, improved living standards, good health and material wealth we now enjoy appear not to have made us happier. Individuals are lonelier and more depressed than ever. Forget being ecstatic or joyful, he says – most of us do not even know how to be at peace.

Sadhguru's ideas are not rocket science, but they touch something primal and human within us. Remember those reflections on the daily sunrise I mentioned in the Introduction? He reminds us that every sunrise is a miracle: not only to gaze at, but as a scientific fact. The sun is the source of energy and life. If it did not rise every morning, within about 18 hours everything would freeze over; plants would be deprived of light and animals of warmth, and eventually the world would end.

Each day around one million people in the world will die: it could be you or someone you love. Every morning that we wake is, in this sense, a miracle: today you are alive, and the world is full of miracles for you to explore. And yet we persist in waking up in a bad mood, feeling grumpy or having 'bad days'. Remember: today you are alive and the cosmos is working in perfect balance – no day should be a bad day.

The Science of Balance

> 66 *When diet is wrong medicine is of no use.*
> *When diet is correct medicine is of no need.* 99
> **Ayurvedic proverb**

Another of these ancient Eastern traditions is Ayurveda. Even if you don't know much about it, you've probably heard of it, along with Ayurvedic terms like 'vata', 'pitta' and 'kapha'. This 5,000-year-old Hindu tradition may seem outdated or irrelevant in our twenty-first century lives but Ayurveda is less complicated and more logical than it might first appear. And it still has plenty to teach us today.

You can think of Ayurveda as the science of balance – and balance is at the heart of your primal journey.

What's the big deal about balance, you might ask? Well, this goes beyond eating your five-a-day and regular exercise: it's about finding balance for your body on a more primal, individual level.

Modern life throws us all sorts of challenges: too much stress, too little sleep, too much food, too little exercise, too much alcohol or caffeine. And there's plenty of evidence that we're feeling out of balance: remember that 400 per cent increase in alleged food allergies? Among all the health scares, product hype and misinformation, it can be hard to listen to what our bodies really need. Even those who are happy, healthy and well-informed about nutrition could be forgiven for getting confused. In a recent report entitled 'Miracle foods, myths and the media' the NHS analysed 344 different news articles. They found that 27 foods were labelled as harmful by journalists, while 65 were declared beneficial, and 14 were labelled both healthy and harmful in different headlines. Chocolate, for example, can reportedly cause weak bones and depression, but other studies have claimed that it can also help to fight cancer. Eggs, grapefruit, caffeine and fish oils were among those substances which were declared both good *and* bad for us! It's no wonder that many of us feel anxious or simply out of balance.

This is where Ayurveda comes in. At the heart of this ancient Vedic science is the notion of a body in balance. In Sanskrit, *ayu* means life and *veda* means science. Ayurveda takes a holistic view of health, treating the individual as a whole, including physical *and* spiritual well-being. It also incorporates yoga and meditation, and even astrology.

Find Your Own Path

The Ayurvedic premise is simple: we all have different body types and therefore different foods agree, or disagree, with us. What is good for one person may not agree with another: you need to experiment with what works for you. Some people feel great on a vegetarian diet, whereas others crave red meat; some feel bloated from wheat, while others can eat bread, pasta and rice without a twinge.

For example, I've experienced severe migraine all my life. The advice from experts was always the same: stay away from red wine, cheese, citrus fruit and dark chocolate. I assumed they were right and avoided these so-called 'trigger foods'. It was only when I started thinking about it that I realised it was making no difference – these weren't triggers for me at all. Red wine didn't bring on a migraine; anxiety did. (As for chocolate, that's definitely part of my diet!)

Ayurveda and Common Sense

Understanding the basic principles of Ayurveda helps you to work out your 'type'. Once you understand a little more about your body, you can stop fighting it or depriving it, and instead start listening to what it needs. Ayurveda takes a common-sense approach to eating and everyday life; it can help you tune into how your body works, what balances or imbalances it and why you might crave certain things.

Ayurveda also allows for individual differences. For decades we've slavishly followed the guidelines that a woman should consume around 2,000 calories, and a man around 2,500 calories, a day. Just like the inaccurate food messages, these generalisations on calories take no account of our activity levels, the food we're eating (all calories are not the same), or our height, age, metabolism or body type. A woman in a sedentary job in her mid-50s will have different energy requirements to an athlete in her 20s. Even our brains need fuel: three-hours of exam revision is hard work, for example, and demands more food than lying on the sofa watching a DVD.

Remember: we're all unique and we all need different amounts of food, rest and exercise.

Key Ayurvedic Principles

- Eat according to your body's personality or 'dosha' (see below).

- Eating according to your dosha will balance the elements: ether, air, fire, water and earth.

- Eat a balance of different tastes or 'rasas'.

- Eat at the right time and in the right way to balance your digestive fire or 'agni'.

- Eat simple combinations of food that are easily digestible.

- Eat seasonally to balance the elements of each season.

All About the Dosha

Your dosha is responsible for all the biological, psychological and physiological functions of your body, mind and consciousness. The three doshas are *vata*, *pitta* and *kapha*. Everyone possesses all three doshas in different proportions – but in general, one type will be dominant, or majority, with another minority type.

- Your dosha is your unique body and personality type.

- Each one of us is born with an inherent combination of doshas.

- Our doshas determine our fundamental constitution or 'prakruti'.

- Your 'prakruti' is the body type you were born with. This never changes, no matter what you do throughout your life: it's your inherent nature.

- Imbalance of the doshas leads to diseases (vikriti).

Determine Your Dosha

In order to determine your dosha, look at the main characteristics of vata, pitta and kapha types. Going through this list, tick each one that applies to you. You may find yourself immediately identifying with one type, or you may feel more balanced between two. (It's rare to be *only* one dosha type.)

Which of the following describes you most accurately?

Vata is predominantly ether and air

Pitta is predominantly fire and water

Kapha is predominantly water and earth

❧ Predominantly vata ❧

Naturally slim with light frame, prominent bones and veins

Loses weight easily with stress or worry, difficulty gaining weight

Often suffers from dry skin and hair, weak nails

Creative or arty interests or work

Restless, fidgety, adventurer, talkative, enthusiastic

Can also be indecisive and excessively anxious

Irregular appetite and eating habits

Occasional gas or bloating, sometimes constipation

Light sleeper (e.g. six hours per night); prefers naps

Feels the cold and has poor circulation; doesn't sweat much

Craves sunshine and warm weather

Tendency to bone and back problems.

❧ Predominantly pitta ❧

Medium frame/constant weight

Loses and gains weight fairly easily

Combination skin and hair, oily and dry in places, lustrous but
sometimes thinning

Sweats a lot

Moderately active, with plenty of energy

Strong appetite and digestion; irritable if hungry

Prone to acidity or heartburn, and also loose bowels

Moderate sleeper (seven hours per night); sleeps soundly
in short bursts

Not a fan of hot sun; prefers shades and uses lots of suncream

Good concentration and decision-making

Makes a great speaker and teacher; ambitious, authoritative and clear

Can be aggressive, short-tempered or argumentative.

🌿 Predominantly kapha 🌿

Strong, heavy or stocky; may find it difficult to lose weight

Radiant skin, shiny hair, strong nails, glossy, grow easily,
can be oily

Sweats moderately

Constant appetite but weaker in the mornings (may skip breakfast)

Occasional heartburn or nausea

Regular daily bowel movements

Heavy sleeper, likes to wake late; feels slow on waking

Can manage weather extremes, but not a fan of
cold/damp weather

Slow movements; can be lazy

Calm, thoughtful, loyal, patient, steady, likes routines,
down to earth

Can be stubborn when stressed, resistant to change, depressive.

This is just a basic introduction to Ayurveda. If you identify with some of these traits, you might want to find out more. A good place to start is *The Body Balance Diet Plan* (by Eminé Ali Rushton) where you can read up on the food which suits your dosha, as well as other Ayurvedic advice. Even if you don't follow all the principles, you can see how it fits into the primal journey you're on. Our emotions, physical and mental health are all affected by our individual temperament and characteristics, just as we're affected by the world around us, by seasons and climate. It's all about eating and living in balance with your type.

Everyday Spirituality

You might be a yoga devotee but find that meditation doesn't work for you; you might feel intrigued by Ayurveda, but less keen on Eastern mysticism. There are no right or wrong paths to finding your primal spirituality. Anything which absorbs you, gives you peace of mind or spiritual nourishment, or simply helps you to find that primal headspace is worth pursuing. Don't ignore your body's instincts for happiness. If something makes you feel joyous, uplifted or refreshed, chances are it will be good for your soul. We could all find opportunities to weave more positive spirituality into our everyday lives.

There are many ways to find your reset button. Switch off your phone for an hour, and try any of the following.

- **Gardening.** Look closely at the plants, touch the earth and the leaves, smell the flowers, do some weeding, pruning or watering. If you're feeling stressed, watching insects and worms in their own little universe can help to put things in perspective! If you don't have a garden, find a park, canal or any local green space.

- **Commune with animals.** Take a dog for a walk, curl up with a cat, watch fish in a pond, or visit a zoo or a city farm. You can even borrow a pet for the weekend; see www.borrowmydoggy.com, for example, a website which matches time-poor dog owners with keen borrowers.

- **Get down with the kids.** Like animals, children help to set things in perspective. Their natural enthusiasm, curiosity and sense of kindness will take you far away from the stresses of adult life. If you don't have children, nephews or nieces, you could offer to babysit for a friend or volunteer with a youth group.

- **Get arty.** Buy a set of watercolours, paint a mural on a wall at home, play with Lego or build a sandcastle.

- **Listen to music.** Lie on the floor (very primal, very grounding) and play your favourite CD or record from beginning to end. No shuffle, no distractions – just listen right through.

- Read a poem or write some 'morning pages'.

- **Learn to dance, take up an instrument or join a choir** – anything difficult and absorbing. You won't have time to worry about work when you're trying to master a new skill.

- **Talk to a friend.** No phones, no other distractions – just the two of you. Try to really listen.

Time to Talk

Talking to others sounds simple, but it can have profound effects. Being close to others is at the root of what it means to be human: talking, listening, laughing, sharing – these are positive, primal experiences. Much of our unhappiness comes from social isolation: in the UK alone, single-person households are set to increase by two million over the next decade. The elderly are particularly vulnerable, with increased life expectancy leaving more of them living alone, widowed, often weak or infirm, and with friends and family too far away for regular visits. Up to 16 per cent of the UK population have social interactions only once a week or less.

Across Europe, inventive new homeshare schemes have been launched to match impoverished students with pensioners who have a spare room to rent out. In return for cheap lodging, the older person gets company and conversation, someone to share meals with and the safety of having someone around. In recession-hit times, with a growing shortage of affordable properties, this could be just the kind of creative social thinking we need. Whether young or old, we all benefit from the daily interactions and shared living.

Something which is positively primal and enjoyable, and leaves you glowing with virtue, is visiting an older person in your neighbourhood. Sometimes called 'befriending', plenty of organisations can organise this, and it can be arranged to suit your schedule. A few years ago I decided to give up one hour per week (the equivalent of a run or a gym class) and I began to visit an old lady called Hilda. It was never just an hour – not because she was demanding, but simply because once we got talking we couldn't stop. We chatted about everything from politics to celebrities to what her life was like growing up the 1930s (and she made delicious lemon drizzle cake).

If you're interested in befriending an older person, check out the following websites:

www.ageuk.org.uk
www.beafriendtoday.org.uk
www.contact-the-elderly.org.uk
www.independentage.org.

Primal Spirituality

Solidarity, gratitude and kindness are the cornerstones of primal spirituality. There are miracles all around, if we only open our eyes. There is deep kindness and compassion within every one of us. The potential for friendship and love is everywhere, too. Total happiness may not be within our grasp, but positivity is. Religious, non-religious or somewhere in between, we can all find a version of primal spirituality on this Earth. Talking, listening and sharing with others, finding activities which absorb us, breathing deeply and practising awareness: these are simple ways to boost our primal joy. Every day, every sunrise, is something to celebrate.

Conclusion

Why Now for Primal? It's clear that the age of information has not been an unmitigated success. The past few decades have seen a flowering of scientific breakthroughs, digital development and global connection, but they have also produced an epidemic of depression, obesity and loneliness. We have learned how to put humans on the Moon and explore other planets, while at the same time damaging our own. We've become increasingly tangled up in virtual reality, caught up in our digital worlds and transfixed by our screens.

Now is the time to learn to reconnect with the world around us, to go beyond the emoticon and the hashtag in our emotional interactions. In the end, this world is all we have. The moment for primal is now, while there are still hedgehogs and skylarks to be saved, books to be read and forests to walk in. Before we lose ourselves in a parallel digital universe, let's remember what's special about this earth, and what it means to be human. Whether it's for the sake of the environment, your own health, your children's future, or a combination of all these reasons, it's time to go primal.

When Not to Go Primal

In general, going primal is a good option – but not every time. Here are a few areas of life where you definitely shouldn't go back to basics.

Sunscreen: after your allotted 15 minutes of sunlight to boost vitamin D levels, it's recommended that you use a daily SPF cream all year round. In strong sunshine you should use a high-quality high-factor sunscreen. Remember: any skin tanning is skin damage. Forget suntans and fake it.

Sex: contraception is one of the great advances of modern life. You should not be playing roulette with your sexual health or risking unwanted pregnancy.

Teeth: don't benefit from primal dental treatment (check out the cavemen!) and neither do feet, unless you want hardened gnarly trotters.

Medicine and other healthcare: for obvious reasons!

In most other areas of your life, from food to fitness, family and relationships, to work and play, your mind and body will benefit from going primal. All it takes is positivity, curiosity and a willingness to try new things.

> 66 *There are some who can live without wild things,*
> *and some who cannot.* 99
> **Aldo Leopold**

I disagree. No matter how far from nature we may live and how busy, urban or digital our lives may be, we all need 'wild things'. No one can truly thrive without fresh air, green space, beauty and silence. Without wildness, we risk forgetting that the sky is full of stars. Without wildness, we risk becoming unhealthy and unhappy in body and soul.

Packed into cities, glued to our screens, plugged in and logged on, we sometimes forget to look around us, touch the people closest to us and smell the spring flowers or autumn bonfires. Despite the damage we've already caused – from deforestation and overfishing to mass extinctions, climate change and global warming – the Earth clings on. The seasons are still changing and the sun is still rising and setting.

Just like our planet, we're resilient. No matter how stressed or depressed we may feel, how burnt out or over-connected we get at times, living primally reconnects us with the world around us. It could be as simple as talking to a friend, walking in the park or swimming in the sea: the sources of primal joy are all around. When we make those conscious efforts to reconnect with our surroundings, we find ourselves more attuned to our emotions and our physical instincts, happier, healthier and closer to nature.

Living more primally means practising kindness and generosity: taking time to care for, and share with, friends and strangers. It means replacing virtual connection with truly meaningful human interaction; disconnecting from the digital world and opening our eyes to the beauty around us. It's about reusing more and wasting less; valuing what we already have rather than trying to get more; treasuring the intangible gifts of love and friendship above money or possessions. Most of all, it's believing that every one of us matters; every individual can make a difference.

An acupuncturist once told me: 'Everything you need, you have.' At times of uncertainty or anxiety, it's a profoundly soothing thought. And in a primal sense, it's true.

However, life is rarely plain sailing. Most of us at some time or another will experience depression or despair, or just a sense of needing to get away from it all – a desire to escape our jobs, our screens, our houses and maybe even those close to us. Remember that whether you live in the countryside or a town, you'll find a refuge in the natural world. Taking time out, being alone, finding space for your own thoughts are all essential. Going primal is grounding, in the most literal sense: walk by a river, gaze at the clouds or just sit quietly in a patch of greenery. When you feel yourself becoming overwhelmed or frazzled by modern life, take five minutes out. Breathe deeply; lie down on the earth. Remember that you belong on this planet. 'Everything you need, you have,' and you're exactly where you need to be.

Living primally makes for a happier and simpler existence. It helps us to reject guilt, shame and fear, and instead live by instinct, joy and kindness. It puts us back in touch with our true selves, and increases our capacity to give and receive joy. Living in a kinder, cleaner, greener way helps us to regain the spring in our step. Remember: your primal nature is already within you. You hold the key to becoming happier and healthier, calmer and stronger. Don't miss out on the daily miracles within and around you: be human, be positive, be primal.

Acknowledgements

Thank you to everyone at Summersdale Publishers, especially Alastair Williams, Claire Plimmer and Lizzie Curtin. To Abbie Headon and Debbie Chapman for their editorial insight and friendship, and to Daniela Nava for her skilful editing.

Thanks to Joanna Tarbit, Nick Breakell, Libby Courtice, Rita Guenigault, Susan Archer, Michael Lee Rattigan, Toby Hardman, Phil Marr, Freda Breakell and Renee McGregor.

Thanks to all the inspiring readers who keep me writing.

To Findlay Wilson, Nana, Marie Schendler and TGW, in loving memory.

Thank you to my siblings, Katie, Philip, Alice and Trim, and my parents Cecil and Jean Woolf.

References

Buettner, Dan *The Blue Zones Solution: Eating and Living Like the World's Healthiest People* (2011, National Geographic)

Curtis, Susan and Johnson, Fran and Thomas, Pat *Neal's Yard Beauty Book* (2015, Dorling Kindersley)

Greenfield, Susan *Mind Change: How digital technologies are leaving their mark on our brains* (2015, Rider)

Hesse, Herman *Siddhartha* (1922, New Directions)

Hilton, Steve *More Human: Designing a World Where People Come First* (2015, WH Allen)

James, Oliver *Affluenza* (2007, Vermilion)

Lawson, Nigella *Kitchen: Recipes from the Heart of the Home* (2010, Chatto & Windus)

Leopold, Aldo *A Sand Country Almanac and Sketches Here and There* (1968, Oxford University Press)

McGregor, Renee *Training Food: Get the Fuel You Need to Achieve Your Goals – Before, During and After Exercise* (2015, Watkins Publishing)

Monbiot, George *Feral: Searching for Enchantment on the Frontiers of Rewilding* (2014, Penguin)

Monbiot, George *Heat: How to Stop the Planet Burning* (2007, Penguin)

Phillips, Roger *Wild Food: A Complete Guide for Foragers* (2014, Macmillan)

Pollan, Michael *In Defence of Food: The Myth of Nutrition and the Pleasures of Eating: An Eater's Manifesto* (2009, Penguin)

Rapley, Chris and Macmillan, Duncan *2071: The World We'll Leave our Grandchildren* (2015, John Murray)

Rew, Kate *Wild Swim* (2009, Guardian Books)

Reynolds, Richard *On Guerrilla Gardening: A Handbook for Gardening Without Boundaries* (2009, Bloomsbury)

Rushton, Eminé Ali *The Body Balance Diet Plan: Lose Weight, Gain Energy and Feel Fantastic with the Science of Ayurveda* (2015, Watkins Publishing)

Slater, Nigel *The Kitchen Diaries (Volumes 1–3)* (2005; 2012; 2015, Fourth Estate)

Toomey, Christine *The Saffron Road: A Journey with Buddha's Daughters* (2015, Portobello Books)

Turkle, Sherry *Alone Together: Why We Expect More From Technology and Less From Each Other* (2013, Basic Books)

Woodhall, Victoria and Sattin, Jonathan *Everyone Try Yoga: Finding your yoga fit in association with Triyoga* (2013, Kyle Books)

Have you enjoyed this book?
If so, why not write a review on your favourite website?

If you're interested in finding out more about our books,
find us on Facebook at **Summersdale Publishers** and
follow us on Twitter at **@Summersdale**.

Thanks very much for buying this Summersdale book.

www.summersdale.com